Childhood Depression

Dante Cicchetti, Karen Schneider-Rosen, *Editors*

NEW DIRECTIONS FOR CHILD DEVELOPMENT
WILLIAM DAMON, *Editor-in-Chief*

Number 26, December 1984

Paperback sourcebooks in
The Jossey-Bass Social and Behavioral Sciences Series

Jossey-Bass Inc., Publishers
San Francisco • Washington • London

Dante Cicchetti, Karen Schneider-Rosen (Eds.).
Childhood Depression.
New Directions for Child Development, no. 26.
San Francisco: Jossey-Bass, 1984.

New Directions for Child Development Series
William Damon, *Editor-in-Chief*

Copyright © 1984 by Jossey-Bass Inc., Publishers
        and
        Jossey-Bass Limited

Copyright under International, Pan American, and Universal
Copyright Conventions. All rights reserved. No part of
this issue may be reproduced in any form—except for brief
quotation (not to exceed 500 words) in a review or professional
work—without permission in writing from the publishers.

New Directions for Child Development (publication number
USPS 494-090) is published quarterly by Jossey-Bass Inc., Publishers.
Second-class postage rates are paid at San Francisco, California,
and at additional mailing offices.

Correspondence:
Subscriptions, single-issue orders, change of address notices, undelivered
copies, and other correspondence should be sent to Subscriptions,
Jossey-Bass Inc., Publishers, 433 California Street, San Francisco
California 94104.

Editorial correspondence should be sent to the Editor-in-Chief,
William Damon, Department of Psychology, Clark University,
Worcester, Massachusetts 01610.

Library of Congress Catalogue Card Number LC 84-81188
International Standard Serial Number ISSN 0195-2269
International Standard Book Number ISBN 87589-986-2

Cover art by Willi Baum
Manufactured in the United States of America

Ordering Information

The paperback sourcebooks listed below are published quarterly and can be ordered either by subscription or single-copy.

Subscriptions cost $35.00 per year for institutions, agencies, and libraries. Individuals can subscribe at the special rate of $25.00 per year *if payment is by personal check*. (Note that the full rate of $35.00 applies if payment is by institutional check, even if the subscription is designated for an individual.) Standing orders are accepted. Subscriptions normally begin with the first of the four sourcebooks in the current publication year of the series. When ordering, please indicate if you prefer your subscription to begin with the first issue of the *coming* year.

Single copies are available at $8.95 when payment accompanies order, and *all single-copy orders under $25.00 must include payment*. (California, New Jersey, New York, and Washington, D.C., residents please include appropriate sales tax.) For billed orders, cost per copy is $8.95 plus postage and handling. (Prices subject to change without notice.)

Bulk orders (ten or more copies) of any individual sourcebook are available at the following discounted prices: 10–49 copies, $8.05 each; 50–100 copies, $7.15 each; over 100 copies, *inquire*. Sales tax and postage and handling charges apply as for single copy orders.

To ensure correct and prompt delivery, all orders must give either the *name of an individual* or an *official purchase order number*. Please submit your order as follows:

Subscriptions: specify series and year subscription is to begin.
Single Copies: specify sourcebook code (such as, CD8) and first two words of title.

Mail orders for United States and Possessions, Latin America, Canada, Japan, Australia, and New Zealand to:
    Jossey-Bass Inc., Publishers
    433 California Street
    San Francisco, California 94104

Mail orders for all other parts of the world to:
    Jossey-Bass Limited
    28 Banner Street
    London EC1Y 8QE

New Directions for Child Development Series
William Damon, *Editor-in-Chief*

CD1 *Social Cognition,* William Damon
CD2 *Moral Development,* William Damon
CD3 *Early Symbolization,* Howard Gardner, Dennie Wolf
CD4 *Social Interaction and Communication During Infancy,* Ina C. Uzgiris
CD5 *Intellectual Development Beyond Childhood,* Deanna Kuhn
CD6 *Fact, Fiction, and Fantasy in Childhood,* Ellen Winner, Howard Gardner

CD7   *Clinical-Developmental Psychology,* Robert L. Selman, Regina Yando
CD8   *Anthropological Perspectives on Child Development,* Charles M. Super,
      Sara Harkness
CD9   *Children's Play,* Kenneth H. Rubin
CD10 *Children's Memory,* Marion Perlmutter
CD11 *Developmental Perspectives on Child Maltreatment,* Ross Rizley, Dante Cicchetti
CD12 *Cognitive Development,* Kurt W. Fischer
CD13 *Viewing Children Through Television,* Hope Kelly, Howard Gardner
CD14 *Childrens' Conceptions of Health, Illness, and Bodily Functions,*
      Roger Bibace, Mary E. Walsh
CD15 *Children's Conceptions of Spatial Relationships,* Robert Cohen
CD16 *Emotional Development,* Dante Cicchetti, Petra Hesse
CD17 *Developmental Approaches to Giftedness and Creativity,*
      David Henry Feldman
CD18 *Children's Planning Strategies,* David Forbes, Mark T. Greenberg
CD19 *Children and Divorce,* Lawrence A. Kurdek
CD20 *Child Development and International Development: Research-Policy Interfaces,*
      Daniel A. Wagner
CD21 *Levels and Transitions in Children's Development,* Kurt W. Fischer
CD22 *Adolescent Development in the Family,* Harold D. Grotevant,
      Catherine R. Cooper
CD23 *Children's Learning in the "Zone of Proximal Development,"*
      Barbara Rogoff, James V. Wertsch
CD24 *Children in Families Under Stress,* Anna-Beth Doyle, Dolores Gold, Debbie S.
      Moscowitz
CD25 *Analyzing Children's Play Dialogues,* Frank Kessel, Artin Göncü.

Contents

Editors' Notes 1
Dante Cicchetti, Karen Schneider-Rosen

Chapter 1. Toward a Transactional Model 5
of Childhood Depression
Dante Cicchetti, Karen Schneider-Rosen
A developmental model that acknowledges the complexity of the phenomenon of depression is necessary to account for vulnerability and resilience to the disorder.

Chapter 2. The Developmental Progression of Depression 29
in Female Children
Judy Garber
A study of changes with age in female children's expression of depressive symptomatology indicates that they are consistent with children's developing capacities within cognitive, linguistic, and socioemotional domains.

Chapter 3. Developmental Stage and the Expression of Depressive 59
Disorders in Children: An Empirical Analysis
Maria Kovacs, Stana L. Paulauskas
Findings are reported from an empirical study of the relationship between cognitive and pubertal development and characteristics of the depressive disorders in clinically referred school-age children.

Chapter 4. Young Offspring of Depressed Parents: A Population 81
at Risk for Affective Problems
Carolyn Zahn-Waxler, E. Mark Cummings, Ronald J. Iannotti,
Marian Radke-Yarrow
Emotional problems in young children with a depressed parent are identified.

Index 107

Editors' Notes

The adoption of a developmental perspective for the study of affective disorders has implications for the description and classification of the disorder, for the understanding of etiology and sequelae, and for therapeutic approaches to prognosis and treatment. Researchers who adopt this approach acknowledge the complexity of the questions that they are addressing and do not limit their inquiry to an application of the models, methods, and analyses that are appropriate for the examination of the disorder in adults alone. Rather, they recognize that it is only when descriptions of affective disorders take into account developmental changes in the integration and organization of social, emotional, and cognitive competencies that a more comprehensive understanding of the etiology and sequelae of affective disorders in childhood will be achieved and that methods for classification, diagnosis, and intervention will be improved.

Adherents of the developmental approach are committed to examining the unique characteristics of affective disorders in childhood and seek to understand the ways in which age-appropriate limitations in cognitive, social, or emotional development may account for differences in the expression of specific symptomatology. Their investigation of etiological factors that may underlie the development of affective disorders considers the early precursors to later forms of affective disorders, while recognizing that limitations in the child's cognitive, emotional, or social abilities may prevent the overt manifestations of specific syndromes until later childhood. Researchers committed to this perspective attempt to understand the ways in which early forms of behavior become hierarchically organized into more complex patterns within developmental systems, the manner in which later modes and functions evolve from earlier prototypes, and the processes by which global and diffuse part functions become integrated into wholes. They try to understand the effects of early experiences on later adaptation, simultaneously considering the individual's current level of functioning and the influence of extraorganismic, environmental factors. Affective disorders are studied not only in terms of how they affect current adaptation, but in terms of how they may impede or delay future developmental progress.

The central theme of this volume is that the adoption of a developmental approach will enhance our understanding of the etiology, course, and sequelae of childhood depressive disorders while providing a framework within which diagnoses can be made and appropriate intervention techniques may be implemented. The understanding of normal developmental theory and research illuminates the critical questions to be addressed and highlights those areas of development that appear to be most vulnerable to an affective disorder. Each chapter represents a commitment to applying a developmental perspective to the conceptualization and examination of affective disorders in childhood.

In Chapter One, we describe what we believe to be the best theoretical framework for understanding vulnerability to depression. Our developmental model permits the researcher or clinician to trace the roots, etiology, and nature of adaptation and maladaptation in children who develop an affective disorder. Moreover, it suggests ways in which compensatory mechanisms may buffer a child against the development of an affective disorder. The model acknowledges a multitude of factors, including individual, familial, social, biological, and environmental variables, that may provide a vulnerability to, or a buffer against, an affective disorder. It contains the transactional, dynamic relation that exists among all of these factors as they impinge on the individual and influence one's vulnerabilities and adaptations during different developmental periods.

In Chapters Two and Three the authors present empirical data that is congruent with this developmental perspective and explore the implications of this approach for the expression of depression at different ages. In Chapter Two, Judy Garber presents the results of a research project designed to address developmental changes in the manifest symptomatology of depression. Her findings suggest that age-appropriate classification and assessment techniques are critical to capturing changes with age in depressive symptoms over the course of development. She discusses the implications of these results for a developmental approach to the diagnosis and classification of childhood depression. In Chapter Three, Maria Kovacs and Stana L. Paulauskas report the results of an empirical examination of the relation between level of cognitive functioning and duration or type of depression in clinically referred school-age children. Specifically, they raise questions with regard to the importance of certain cognitive capacities presumed to be critical to the overt manifestations of particular symptoms of depression.

Finally, in the last chapter, Carolyn Zahn-Waxler, E. Mark Cummings, Ronald J. Iannotti, and Marian Radke-Yarrow present empirical data that reflects the application of the developmental approach to the study of children at risk for developing affective disorders. They explore individual differences in the nature and modulation of emotional expressions and in the early social functioning of young children of manic-depressive and unipolar depressed parents. They examine the ways in which coping strategies and affective styles influence the vulnerability to the development of emotional problems in these populations of children.

These chapters illustrate that a developmental approach provides a framework for formulating theoretical and research questions concerning the coherence of development in children with an affective disorder. Together, they acknowledge the complexity of the affective disorders and provide a basis for designing future studies of the processes of adaptation or maladaptation in children who suffer from, or who are at risk for developing, an affective disorder.

Dante Cicchetti
Karen Schneider-Rosen
Editors

Dante Cicchetti is the Norman Tishman Associate Professor of Psychology and Social Relations at Harvard University. His research interests lie in the areas of developmental psychopathology, affective disorders, child maltreatment, socioemotional development, and the neurosciences.

Karen Schneider-Rosen is an assistant professor in the Department of Psychology at Boston College. Her research interests lie in the areas of developmental psychopathology, childhood depression, child maltreatment, and social and emotional development.

A developmental model for conceptualizing vulnerability to childhood depression must consider the multiple transactions among environmental forces, caregiver characteristics, and child characteristics.

Toward a Transactional Model of Childhood Depression

Dante Cicchetti
Karen Schneider-Rosen

There has been a proliferation of interest in the concept of childhood depression since the publication of Rie's (1966) comprehensive review of the literature on the topic. Theoretical and empirical advances have been made in the understanding of the epidemiology, diagnostic criteria, etiology, psychobiology, and treatment of the depressive disorders in childhood (see Kashani and others, 1981). The vast majority of empirical work on childhood depression has incorporated the research and diagnostic tools and the theoretical models that are prevalent in the study of adult dysfunction. Thus, these studies have proceeded by extending to children results, procedures, methods, and theories that have been useful for understanding adult depression. However, as yet there is no theoretical framework within which unity

---

The writing of this chapter was supported by a grant from the National Institute of Mental Health (1-RO1-MH37960-01).
We would like to extend our appreciation and gratitude to Ellen Bressler, Philip Holzman, Joseph Lipinski, Paul Meehl, and Michael Pakaluk. Finally, we wish to thank Ellen Bressler for typing this manuscript.

and conceptual clarity may be brought to the diverse perspectives represented in the study of depression in childhood.

There is considerable controversy about several issues that are crucial to the formulation of a comprehensive theory of childhood depression. Confusion exists over the essential symptoms necessary for diagnosing the disorder, about the way in which depression manifests itself during childhood, about the psychological and psychobiological mechanisms that underlie its occurrence, and about the effect of depressive disorder in childhood on future adaptation. It is unclear whether depression should be viewed as a transient sign of adjustment, as a symptom that is secondary to another illness, or as a syndrome that includes various signs of dysphoric affect. Furthermore, we need to know whether a diagnosis of depression should depend on the subjective, objective, or combined evaluation of discomfort, and who is the most competent and appropriate person to make such an assessment.

While there has been a burgeoning interest in the study of childhood depression in recent years, there are many issues relevant to its investigation that have not been adequately addressed. It appears to be appropriate to integrate and modify what is known about adult depression when exploring childhood depression. However, while existing research and theory relating to adult models of specific pathological disorders can provide important clues for how to approach deviations in childhood, there are several important reasons to apply a developmental orientation to the study of childhood problems.

The Usefulness of a Developmental Approach

The study of childhood depression poses unique problems and raises important research questions. Therefore, it would be unwise to apply results and theories concerning adults too inflexibly when studying depressed children. In particular, a developmental perspective can lead to advances in the study of symptomatology, etiology, sequelae, and biological correlates (Cicchetti and Schneider-Rosen, in press). Current research has not distinguished adequately the developmental considerations that must be made when examining a population of depressed children. For example, current researchers, by consensus, employ Research Diagnostic Criteria (RDC) (Spitzer and others, 1978) or Diagnostic and Statistical Manual-III (DSM-III; American Psychiatric Association, 1980) criteria as a means of isolating a homogeneous group of depressed children. However, these diagnostic formulations were developed based on clinical observations of, and research on, adults (see Puig-Antich, 1980) and are currently employed with adults. We have elsewhere suggested that the board criteria of RDC or DSM-III, although useful for adults, need to be translated into age-appropriate guidelines for children, sensitive to developmental changes in the children's experience and expression of depression (Cicchetti and Schneider-Rosen, in press). Similarly, preliminary studies of possible biological correlates of childhood depression and of the response to insulin induced hypoglycemia (Puig-Antich and others, markers identified in adult depression and psychotropic drugs used with success in adults. Thus, for example, depressed children, like depressed adults, have been reported to hypersecrete cortisol (Puig-Antich and others, 1979), to hyposecrete growth hormone (GH) in response to insulin induced gypoglycemia (Puig-Antich and others, 1984), and to respond to tricyclic medications (Puig-Antich and others, 1979; Puig-Antich and Gittelman, 1982). While these findings may have important implications for understanding biological substrates of depression, there may be particular characteristics that have not been examined in childhood depression due to the reliance upon investigating those factors that have proven to be relevant to adult depression.

A developmental approach is likewise important for understanding the etiology of depression. A number of etiological factors, drawn primarily from the causal theories extant in the study of adult depression (see Akiskal and McKinney, 1975), have been implicated in childhood depression. There are models based on biochemistry, genetics, cognitive distortion, learned helplessness, and behavioral reinforcement. However, developmental differences between children and adults may have implications for the forms that pathological processes take. In particular, it would seem especially important to examine the cognitive developments that may be necessary preconditions for the operation of particular pathological processes. For example, we have proposed that the transition from preoperational to concrete operational thought may be a necessary precondition for the possibility of children making internal and stable causal attributions to themselves, thus making possible an entrenched state of learned helplessness. We have also suggested that certain cognitive changes are also necessary for children to be vulnerable to loss of self-esteem and to pervasive guilt feelings (Cicchetti and Schneider-Rosen, in press). In addition, a developmental approach to the etiology of childhood depression may prepare the way for the formulation of etiological processes that are specific to childhood depression alone.

Our understanding of the sequelae of childhood depression may be deepened through attention to developmental changes. Particularly important, when assessing the impact of depression upon later development, is the notion of *competence* and the role that early competence plays in realizing later competence (Cicchetti and Schneider-Rosen, in press). Following Waters and Sroufe (1983), we can define competence as the ability to utilize environmental and personal resources to attain a satisfactory, age-appropriate adaptation. A child attains such adaptation who successfully resolves the developmental tasks salient to his or her age. Thus, for example, a salient task for the young infant is homeostatic regulation; for the infant between six months and one year old it is the formulation of a secure attachment relationship with primary caregivers; for the toddler major developmental tasks are exploration and mastery of the environment and attainment of autonomy (Waters and Sroufe, 1983). Similar stage-salient tasks can be formulated through the development of formal operations (Cicchetti and Schneider-Rosen, in press). It then becomes important to consider what impact a depressive episode may have according to the age at which it occurs. Its impact, we suggest, works in two ways. First, the depressed child is incompetent throughout the duration of the depressive episode, and this incompetence may in turn play a role in the precipitation of a later episode of depression. Second, since early competence may be predictive of later competence, the early incompetence resulting from the depression may result in later incompetence, which may in turn be a vulnerability factor in the development of a later depressive episode. We may expect that the ramifications that an early episode of depression can have for later development and especially for later depression are related to the developmental time of the earlier depression. Thus, the time of onset of a depressive episode may have specific implications for treatment and future prophylaxis.

A developmental understanding of childhood depression will no doubt become more articulated as knowledge of normal development increases, since pathology can be understood only in the light of normal development (Cicchetti, 1984; Cicchetti and Pogge-Hesse, 1982; Cicchetti and Schneider-Rosen, 1984; Sroufe and Rutter, 1984). In particular, since depression having the florid symptomatology of bipolar depression (that is, manic-depressive illness) is rarer throughout childhood in general (Rutter, in press; but see Sylvester and others, 1984), it is especially important to investigate prototypical forms of adult depression or mania (see, for example, Gaensbauer, 1980; Gaensbauer and others, 1984; Zahn-Waxler and others, 1984; Zahn-Waxler and others, 1984). Since these cannot be detected by available forms of assessment, however, this investigation must await the more precise delineation of diagnostic criteria and the creation of instruments specifically developed for use with children. A knowledge of normal development is also necessary for detecting subtle, psychological differences that may indicate an underlying genetic diathesis for depression. Meehl (1962, 1972) has postulated that the genetic diathesis for *schizophrenia,* which, he argues, is the integrative neural defect of *schizotaxia,* leads ultimately, through a process of social learning, to the development of a schizotypic personality. He suggests that finer methods of assessing *schizotypy* are crucial for the determination of the mode of genetic transmission of schizotaxia and for the discovery of possible well-state or trait makers of schizotaxia (Meehl, 1972, 1978). It seems reasonable to expect that, for some forms of depression, at least, there may be analogues to Meehl's schizotaxia, schizotypy, and schizophrenia. If this is the case, then a better knowledge of normal development could lead to the detection of "depressotypy" in its early forms in young children, which not only may aid in the formulation of theories of transmission and in the discovery of well-state markers, but may also guide intervention and early prophylaxis.

The study of depression from a developmental perspective can make many significant contributions to our theory of normal development, primarily by contributing greater precision to existing theory and by forcing us to examine theories of development critically in relation to our knowledge about psychopathology. The results of such empirical and theoretical investigations may be the description of alternative developmental pathways that lead to the same or different outcomes of the developmental sequence and a weighting of the respective roles of biological, social, emotional, and cognitive factors in mental growth. Furthermore, before one is capable of identifying deviances that exist in a system, one must possess an accurate description of the system itself. Only when we understand the total ongoing development of normal systems can we fully comprehend developmental deviations as adaptational irregularities of those systems (Von Bertalanffy, 1968). Since developmental change may be rapid or gradual, it is necessary to consider normative trends of developing skills in the social, emotional, and cognitive domains so as to be in a better position to evaluate deviation or maladjustment as compared to other children. In addition, it is critical to consider intra-individual variation in the overt manifestations of a depressive episode and individual protective factors or stressors that may inhibit or potentiate depression.

It is impossible to develop cogent, sophisticated diagnoses and treatment plans for depressed children without an appropriate developmental perspective that provides a framework within which vulnerabilities, strengths, or symptoms can be identified. One would not expect to find behavioral isomorphism in the observed signs or symptoms of depression in children of different ages. In addition, one would not predict that the developmental variations in internal cognitive structures would enable children of different ages to employ similar strategies to interpret, express, or defend against their affective experiences or internal emotional states. Thus, a developmental perspective is needed to highlight the processes or symptoms most likely to contribute to vulnerabilities at each developmental level. A developmental scheme is also necessary for tracing the roots, etiology, and nature of maladaptation so that treatment interventions may be planned appropriately. Moreover, a developmental perspective will prove useful for uncovering the level of compensatory mechanisms employed in the face of specific deficiencies.

These considerations indicate that what is needed for the study of childhood depression is (1) a framework that is developmental in nature and that is adequate for both normal and pathological development, and (2) a model, formulated within this framework, that can serve as a basis on which the genetic, neurobiological, constitutional, psychological, familial, environmental, and sociological factors relevant to depression can be analyzed with respect to their interaction with the cognitive, affective, and social domains. We believe that the kind of theoretical perspective suitable for this task is the "organizational" or "organismic" view of development; furthermore, we think that the kind of model most useful for childhood depression is a transactional one. In the remainder of this chapter, we shall first explain what the organizational perspective is; then, we shall propose the outline of a transactional model for the etiology of childhood depression, contrasting it with other kinds of models. It should of course be noted that the findings on childhood depression are currently too incomplete to allow for the formulation of a fully delineated model. The value of what we propose here is largely heuristic: We think that this model can provide an overarching, integrating framework from which one can conceptualize the causes of childhood depression.

The Organizational Approach to Psychopathology

We believe that development may best be understood as a series of structural reorganizations among the cognitive, affective, and social systems of behavior that proceeds by means of differentiation and hierarchical integration (Werner, 1948; Werner and Kaplan, 1963). The relationship between the relatively immature person and the relatively mature one is the relationship between a state of globality and lack of articulation and a state of greater differentiation, articulation, and complexity, effectively organized into hierarchical systems and subsystems (Miller, 1978; Von Bertalanffy, 1968; Werner, 1948). A distinction can thus be drawn between chronological age and developmental age, where the latter is determined by the individual's state of articulation and hierarchical integration.

Given this understanding of development, it is clear that normality may not be conceived merely as conformity to the mean, since we may no more expect that the mean defines normal or healthy development than we can expect that the mean among physiological parameters defines health in organic medicine. Rather, normal development must be seen in terms of structural changes among the child's behavioral systems that reflect the dynamic interactions of changing familial, social, and environmental variables, and, given the absence of extraordinary environmental conditions, allow the child to attain competence. In contrast, psychopathology may be understood as a lack of effective organization among behavioral domains that leads to personal distress and cognitive, affective, or social incompetence. This lack of organization between behavioral systems could represent manifestations either of a failure to achieve a particular level of competence within one behavioral system or the incomplete resolution of certain developmental tasks within a behavioral system (Cicchetti and Schneider-Rosen, in press). When psychopathology is conceptualized in this manner, it becomes crucial to identify the specific developmental arrests or the unsuccessfully resolved developmental tasks implicated in a depressive episode, the environmental stressors involved, and the familial circumstances that may have interfered with the resolution of the developmental issues. Furthermore, it is essential to characterize depression in terms of specific forms of nonintegration, in such a way as to distinguish it from other forms of psychopathology, each of which leaves its own fingerprint of incompetence by leading to peculiar patterns of maladaptation.

The Orthogenetic Principle. The principle that development proceeds from global and diffuse states, by means of differentiation and integration, to states of articulation and hierarchical complexity, is known as the *orthogenetic principle* (Werner, 1948). There are several consequences of this principle for the study of psychopathology in general and childhood depression in particular. First, because development must be viewed in terms of integration and qualitative reorganization rather than mere accretion or expansion, one should not expect behavioral isomorphism in depressive symptomatology across developmental levels. Second, the significance of a behavior in the depressive syndrome must be inferred from the context in which it occurs. This may be called the principle of *holism,* and it derives from the fact that the same function in an organized behavioral system can be fulfilled by two dissimilar behaviors, whereas the same kind of behavior may serve two different functions (Werner and Kaplan, 1963). Similarly, the same behavior may also play different roles in different behavioral domains. This implies that a study of the development of depression and depressive symptomatology is likely to be fruitful, and to reveal the relationship between the pathological process and normal development, only if the behavior of the depressed child is examined simultaneously at the molar and molecular levels (see Cicchetti and Schneider-Rosen, in press). At the molar level broad patterns of organization appear, whereas at the molecular level we see those behavioral units that have been integrated into molar structures. Moreover, those studies of childhood depression that rely on frequency counts alone or that merely list symptoms seen at various ages are not likely to be of great significance for a developmental theory of childhood depression. A third consequence of the orthogenetic principle is that the study of individual differences becomes not merely helpful, but actually essential for an understanding of pathological development.

The orthogenetic principle subsumes several concepts that should be embodied in an adequate model of childhood depression. The first of these is the distinction between *process* and *outcome*. Applying the principle of holism, with its insistence on attention to context, different processes can underlie the same outcome and different outcomes may in some circumstances result from similar processes. This situation highlights the importance of considering multiple pathways to maladaptation, incompetence, and pathology. An adequate model of childhood depression must be able to delineate these multiple pathways and to account for their interrelationship. Thus, it is possible that a developmental organization that occurs in particular ecological circumstances may lead to later maladaptation, when ecological conditions change. For example, the securely attached infant in a warm and loving environment and the physically abused infant who avoids contact both have adaptive strategies (Schneider-Rosen and others, in press). They illustrate two separate pathways to early adaptation; however, children using an avoidance strategy with their parents tend to adopt interpersonal strategies that are maladaptive when entering into relations among their peer group (George and Main, 1979).

A model of childhood depression should also incorporate the notion of *microgenesis*. Microgenesis describes the development inherent in psychological processes or events of brief duration. That is, certain processes or events that appear to be static and uniform may actually display a development from globality and diffuseness to articulation and hierarchical integration. Examples of potentially microgenetic processes are perception, recognition, encoding in problem solving, recall, and also transient emotions such as surprise and shock. Microgenesis may play various roles in psychopathology. It may figure in the etiology of disorder: For example, the cognitive distortions that constitute the depressed child's front line of contact with the environment may display a disordered microgenetic structure. In addition, it may be relevant to various defenses employed by the depressed child when coping with depressed mood or depressogenic schemata.

With the increasing differentiation and integration that constitute development also come a greater flexibility and an ability to use substitute means for attaining the same end. (This last point is an additional reason why the context principle characterizes development.) But the greater flexibility of the more developed individual does not consist solely in the horizontal ability to substitute various relatively refined strategies for one another. It also consists in an ability to use flexibly various models of behavior that were available at earlier points of development and that have since been incorporated into the hierarchy. This ability to draw upon strategies that have become incorporated into a more encompassing structural organization in the course of development may be referred to as *hierarchical motility*. It is an ability to choose from a vertical array of alternative means to an end. Hierarchical motility seems to be crucial for normal growth and development. Problem solving, creative processes, and coping strategies may first do away with differentiations in a limited domain by means of hierarchical motility, then proceed to make new differentiations and integration within this domain, but now particularly suited to dealing effectively with the problem or difficulty that occasioned this response. It is here that Piaget's (1952) concepts of assimilation and accommodation as two different strategies with respect to environmental problems, obstacles, or insults may find their most direct application in an organizational model. Novel differentiation and hierarchical integration represent accommodation if the structure of the integration is adapted to that of the problem, obstacle, or insult; they represent assimilation, however, if their effect is to change or to remove difficulty.

These two processes of adaptation underline the way in which a hierarchically organized and developing person may display "directedness" or "self-righting" tendencies (Sameroff and Chandler, 1975; Waddington, 1966). The capacity to respond with resilience to environmental changes, threats, and insults is typical of systems that embody complex, hierarchically organized homeostatic systems. Kaplan's (1966) "polarities of orthogenesis" may be helpful here in characterizing either pathological states or conditions that may constitute a vulnerability to depression. The first polarity is that of rigid versus flexible. The rigid individual cannot employ assimilation or accommodation to adapt to environmental challenges, whereas the flexible individual can. The second polarity, labile versus stable, refers to the degree to which the flexible person can retain integrity in the midst of adaptations. The labile person undergoes extreme changes in psychological structure in response to relatively transient or minor environmental fluctuation, while the stable individual displays more balanced and orderly strategies in dealing with the environment. It should be noted that, although these polarities have a somewhat abstract and arid air when they are considered on the strictly theoretical plane, when they are actually manifested in the psychological structure of a developing child they can cause the greatest distress and mental pain. If, following Sandler and Joffe (1965), we define mental pain as a reaction to a perceived discrepancy between an ideal state and the actual one, it is apparent that both rigidity and lability may result in a great deal of suffering. The structurally rigid child will exhibit frustration and anger in the fact of an inability to adjust to changing environmental exigencies; the structurally labile child may lose self-esteem and sense his or her inability to order or control the environment.

Behavioral Systems. The notion of a behavioral system is postulated to explain observed patterns among discrete, individual behaviors (see, for example, Ainsworth, 1973; Bischof, 1975; Bowlby, 1969). There is strong theoretical support from three different disciplines for the postulation of such systems. In ethology, investigators conceive of the variety of animal behaviors used for such different purposes as food gathering, mating, territorial defense, aggression, and dominance sorting in terms of different, hierarchically organized systems. In ethology, the notion of behavioral system replaces unclear notions such as drive or instinct; in psychology, it can serve to illuminate traditional concepts such as faculties and more current ones such as the metapsychological structures employed in Freudian psychology. In neurophysiology, the central nervous system has been found to have a hierarchical structure. It seems natural to assume a behavioral analogue or manifestation. Finally, computer science and control systems theory indicate that a hierarchically organized system, which uses servo-mechanisms and homeostatic regulation, may best simulate the goal-directed activity seen in living organisms. From this one may assume as a working hypothesis that the human psyche has a similar structure.

Psychopathology can be viewed as a lack of integration among behavioral systems. The effects and consequences of lags and advances in a behavioral system in relation to other systems—not merely the developmental immaturity of a system—are of particular importance for a model of childhood depression.

A Transactional Model

Review of Relevant Proposals. There are basically four models that have been proposed in the past as conceptualizations of psychopathology: the *early experience, main-effects, diathesis-stress,* and *vulnerability* models. The last two of these have been formulated especially for adult schizophrenia, but they can easily be adjusted for application to adult depression. However, the adjustments that need to be made in all of these models in order to apply them to childhood depression are not trivial, and, in fact, the model that results when development is adequately accounted for is a *transactional* model, which differs significantly from the four listed above.

The early experience and main-effects models are too simplistic for most of today's investigators. An early experience model charges that later psychopathology is determined almost solely by some childhood experience that lies dormant for some period of time before finally making itself apparent in the form of psychopathology. The main-effects model is similar, though it does not limit the action of the aggravating cause of psychopathology to early experience in childhood. According to the main-effects model, psychopathology is the direct and inevitable result of some specific early pathogenic experience or process that exerts a profound impact on the individual throughout the life span. For example, within the study of depression, researchers-employing the early experience model would focus on uncovering the early experiential factors that may render a child vulnerable to developing an affective disorder later in life—for example, perceived or real loss of a significant love object in infancy or early childhood (Bowlby, 1980). Both the early experience model and the main-effects model can easily be seen to be deficient for several reasons. First, they posit a strict cause-effect determinism that is in fact neither seen in clinical experience nor supported by experimental work. Second, they ignore the importance of the person's active response to the agent that is supposed to lead to pathology. Third, they do not explain variations in duration before the outbreak of pathology or the role of later factors in determining form, content, and severity of pathology. Fourth, efforts directed only to identifying the early experiences that predispose an individual to depression later in life negate the importance and value of examining experiences that occur throughout the life span that may either interact with earlier experiences and mediate against their potentially negative impact, or create new vulnerabilities that may result in more severe pathology.

Few researchers or theorists would assent to such simplistic models of psychopathology; nonetheless, a surprisingly large number of studies have been carried out that seem to have been designed in accordance with these models. From a theoretical or conceptual point of view, however, the diathesis-stress model is currently perhaps the most widely accepted model of psychopathology. The diathesis-stress model was originally proposed to explain how a genetic predisposition may be a necessary but not sufficient condition for the development of schizophrenia (Gottesman and Shields, 1972). Concerning the genetic diathesis, there are two possibilities: It may be either mono- or polygenic. If the diathesis is monogenic, then the predisposition for psychopathology is an all-or-nothing affair—one either has the predisposition or not. However, what determines why some persons with the predispoistion develop schizophrenia and others do not depends on various potentiating and compensatory factors, some of which concern the individual (for example, personality structure, cognitive set) and others of which concern the environment (for example, family structure, life events). According to the monogenic theory, there may be additional polygenic determination of some of these potentiating and compensatory factors, namely, the physiological, biochemical, and psychological characteristics of the individual and his or her family. According to the hypothesis of a polygenic diathesis, the predisposition to develop psychopathology may itself vary in degree, depending upon the number of relevant genes one inherits and their interactions. And, this diathesis, too, can be potentiated or compensated by a variety of factors, some of which may also be under varying degrees of genetic control.

Where does the "stress" part enter in, in the diathesis-stress distinction? In its more sophisticated form (Meehl, 1972), the diathesis-stress model is not really what its name indicates, and, in fact, approximates what we refer to as a transactional model. The common understanding of the relationship between diathesis and stress is cruder than the explanation in the preceding paragraph. Psychopathology is held to be a function of two variables: an initial, unchanging genetic inheritance and environmental stressors. The interaction between these factors is held to be additive: The diathesis places a person at one of several degrees of risk, and all that is required to put that person over a temporally invariant threshold for pathology is a certain amount of environmental stress. Moreover, according to this simplistic diathesis-stress model, the result of this interaction between diathesis and stress at one point in time does not enter into the determination of the person's condition at a later point. Clearly, however, this discontinuity is unsatisfactory. What we should like to see in our model of psychopathology is the person's state at one point in time (biochemical effects, psychological organization, cognitive style, motivational set, and so on) as well as the state of the person's environment (family organization and dynamics, interpersonal relationships, psycho-ecology in the workplace, and so on) also entering into the determination of the person's state at a later point, along with genetic diathesis and stress.

For this reason the *vulnerability* model (Zubin and Spring, 1977) of pyschopathology represents a real advance over a simple diathesis-stress, interactional model. It approaches being a truly transactional model. According to this model, vulnerability to a particular disorder is actually a distinct construct, orthogonal to competence and to motivational factors. Vulnerability is not seen as a constant, determined solely by a genetic endowment; rather, it increases or decreases according to the type and severity of stressors experienced, the person's perception of those stressors, and various constitutional and ecological factors. Moreover, these factors can interact synergistically so that potentiating and compensatory factors can increase or decrease vulnerability according to their patterns of interaction.

As helpful as this approach is, the vulnerability model suffers from two fundamental difficulties. First, it is unclear whether vulnerability ought to be treated as a construct, analogous to competence or types of motivation, such as "coping effort." The trouble with the vulnerability model is that it posits a specific vulnerability for schizophrenia. There is nothing in the model to hinder its application to other disorders, and indeed, it seems reasonable to presume that a similar model could be formulated for every diagnostic category in a psychiatric nosology. But it would not be parsimonious to postulate a different vulnerability model for each form of psychopathology. Moreover, disorder-specific constructs of vulnerability would play no role in an explanation of normal development. If one considers analogies taken from organic medicine, this point becomes clearer. Although there are risk factors for various forms of pathology, and one can even quantify morbid risk, it would be neither meaningful nor helpful to attempt to characterize human physiology in terms of vulnerabilities corresponding to specific pathologies.

The second problem with the vulnerability model is determining the threshold of vulnerability beyond which stress produces illness. According to the vulnerability model, stress can either precipitate an episode of pathology or else render the person more vulnerable. However, the question arises of what factors determine what this threshold is. It seems natural to conclude that a combination of constitutional, psychological, biological, and environmental factors determine it. If that is so, then the same factors determine both vulnerability and the threshold distinguishing the vulnerable but healthy person from the sick person. It then seems that vulnerability amounts to no more than degree of wellness. An alternative understanding of the vulnerability model would state that the genetic endowment determines the threshold of illness. On this interpretation, however, the vulnerability model then reduces to an interactional, diathesis-stress model.

Retracing our steps for a moment, we can say that these problems with the vulnerability model stem from an error concerning the logic of dispositions (Carnap, 1936; Pap, 1958; Sellars, 1958). Vulnerability is a dispositional concept, and, like all such concepts, it implies that a given state will result when an event of a particular kind occurs. In the vulnerability model of schizophrenia, we can say that vulnerability is the capacity to develop schizophrenia given the occurrence of some event (or group or constellation of events). However, if one takes vulnerability to denote a disposition, it is then a mistake to hypostatize it, quantify it, and argue that when vulnerability reaches a certain degree of "strength," then illness somehow occurs. In arguing this way, one no longer conceives of a vulnerability as a disposition, but rather as a state or characteristic of the individual, such as "degree of illness" or "degree of wellness." It is true that a disposition can (metaphorically) vary in strength; but when we say that a person is very vulnerable or not very vulnerable to developing an illness, we do not make a statement about the so-called construct of vulnerability, as if it were some trait of the individual; rather, we are indicating what kinds of events must occur to precipitate that state to which the individual is vulnerable in the first place.

A Sketch of a Transactional Model. Reseachers and theoreticians have begun to conceive of children's developmental outcomes as having many historical and causal determinants rather than single-factor etiologies. Since research in the area of childhood depression is firmly rooted in medicine, biology, and the medical model, it is perhaps understandable why the majority of research in the area has focused upon uncovering the symptom characteristics and the biological factors that influence the expression of the symptoms. However, most theoretical depictions of the medical model are simplistic, since biology is a dynamic discipline (Engel, 1977). A true biological or medical model of childhood depression would attribute the occurrence of the psychopathological syndrome to a system breakdown in the dynamic organism-environment transaction (Von Bertalanffy, 1968).

Sameroff and Chandler (1975) have proposed a biological model which is transactional in that it takes into account the interrelations among dynamic systems and the processes characterizing system breakdown. Moreover, they explain the mechanisms by which compensatory, self-righting tendencies (Waddington, 1966) are initiated whenever higher level monitors detect deviations in a subsystem. Thus, a transactional model views the multiple transactions among environmental forces, caregiver characteristics, and child characteristics, as dynamic, reciprocal contributions to the events and outcomes of child development. This model decries the efficacy of simple, linear "cause-effect" models of causality and suggests that it is impossible to understand a child's development by focusing on single pathogenic events. Rather, Sameroff and Chandler (1975) argue that it is necessary to analyze the ways in which the environment responds to a particular child's characteristics at a particular point in time.

The transactional model presents the environment and child as exerting a mutual influence on each other in a dynamic fashion. Therefore, if a child exhibits deviant patterns of development at a specific point in time, it is presumed that it is necessary to consider the environmental characteristics that may be influencing the child's current level of adaptation. If the child demonstrates deviations in the developmental process over time, then it may be assumed that the child has been involved in a continuous maladaptive process (see Sroufe, 1979). The implication of the transactional model is that the continued manifestation of maladaptation depends on environmental support, while the child's characteristics, reciprocally, partially determine the nature of the environment. Consequently, an all-encompassing and theoretically meaningful model of development must yield a formulation of the developmental process that can embrace both stability and change. It must transcend the linear cause-effect models and be complex enough to reflect the multifaceted ways in which constitutional, organismic, and environmental factors transact to affect development.

Risk Factors. The application of a transactional model of development to the etiology of depression requires that one considers the specific risk factors associated with the disorder. A scheme for characterizing the processes involved in a depressive episode must integrate all the factors that have been implicated in the etiology of depression (see Table 1). These factors may be seen to comprise a vulnerability to depression as opposed to resilience to depressive disorder in those children who possess the risk factors for depression. Each outcome—depression or resilience to depressive disorder—may be accounted for in light of those enduring or transient influences that either increase or decrease the probability of the occurrence of a depressive episode. The

Table 1. A Transactional Model of Risk Factors Associated with Childhood Depression

Potentiators Vulnerability	Compensators Protective
1. *Individual* Excessive need for reinforcement Unsuccessful resolution of stage-salient developmental tasks Structuralized negative schemata of self and world Nutritional deficiency Excessive seriousness, whiny, clingy Embryonic phobias, hypochondriasis Failure to individuate Distorted cognitive set Repeated experiences of non-contingency between action and outcome that result in learned helplessness Diminished number of biogenic amines Depressive genotype Offspring of parent(s) with an affective disorder hypersensitivity to frustration Moodiness Poor self-control	1. *Individual* Resiliency to stress Prior experience with stressful events Ability to utilize aggression adaptively Capacity to tolerate disparity between ideal and actual self Successful resolution of stage-salient developmental tasks Availability of defense mechanisms Capacity to conceptualize and differentiate multiple emotions Good physical health/resistance to illness High hedonic capacity Good temperament High threshold for frustration Parents have no prior history of an affective disorder
2. *Familial* Early separation Early loss Pathological, gloomy, depressed parents Manipulative syndrome in parents Early spoiling followed by later rejection Rejection and depreciation by parents Ambivalent attachment Presence of several young children in the home, lack of full-time or part-time employment, absence of a confidant or partner, and loss of mother by separation or death before the age of eleven	2. *Familial* Secure attachment bond to parents History of good parenting and socialization Sibling attachments
3. *Social* Investment of self-esteem in	3. *Social* Good peer relations

Table 1. A Transactional Model of Risk Factors Associated with Childhood Depression (continued)

Potentiators *Vulnerability*	*Compensators* *Protective*
Social (continued) dominant other	*Social (continued)* Availability of social support network
4. *Environmental* Early deprivation Noncontingent negative reinforcement	4. *Environmental* Availability of economic resources Availability of community resources Help from extended family
Challengers	*Buffers*
1. *Individual* Cognitive distortions Stress induced changes in neurochemistry Lack of social supports Ineffective coping style	1. *Individual* Realistic cognitions Use of defense mechanisms Supportive social network
2. *Familial* Loss of ambivalently loved object Bereavement	2. *Familial* Continuation of daily routine Parents responsive to each other and child
3. *Social* Stress specific to negative schemata Situation specific to earlier noncontingent reinforcement	3. *Social* Continuation of daily routine Supportive relations with peers and others
4. *Environmental* Situation specific to earlier noncontingent reinforcement	4. *Environmental* Absence of discord in the home Pleasurable activities

factors associated with each outcome are classified into two broad categories: *Potentiating factors* increase the probability of manifesting a depressive episode, while *compensatory factors* increase the likelihood of remaining resilient. *Transient factors* refer to those influences that are fluctuating and relatively short-lived in duration, whereas *enduring factors* represent more permanent attributes or conditions. Potentiating factors may exert an enduring or transient influence in the development of childhood depression, in the form of individual, familial, social, and environmental factors. Likewise, compensatory factors of a similar nature may be instrumental in bringing about either an enduring or transient resilience to the development of childhood depression.

Within this transactional model of the risk factors associated with childhood depression, *vulnerability factors* include those relatively enduring characteristics of the child, the family, and the social environment that have been identified as playing a significant etiological role in depression. *Challengers* represent more transient factors that could trigger a depressive episode.

The compensatory factors that increase resilience to a depressive disorder even in those children who possess the risk factors for depression include both the enduring influence of protective factors and the transient impact of buffers. *Protective factors* represent conditions that may be psychological, biological, situational, or sociological/cultural. *Buffers* are relatively transient in nature, but may serve to protect the child or the caregiver during periods of unexpected stress. Some examples of vulnerability factors, challengers, protective factors, and buffers, drawn from the theoretical and empirical literature on childhood depression, are presented in Table 1.

It is important to observe the relation between development and the factors relevant for a transactional model. For enduring factors, be they vulnerability or protective factors, developmental changes may be a necessary precondition for their operation (for example, the ability to conceptualize multiple emotions, a protective factor, is made possible by a cognitive change). We can expect transient factors to be age specific. That is, what constitutes a challenge will vary with developmental level, as will what constitutes a buffer.

We may expect a coordination among compensatory and protective factors. This, perhaps, follows from the "self-righting" characteristic of development (Sameroff and Chandler, 1975; Waddington, 1966). For example, with the development of concrete operations the child can make causal attributions to the self (vulnerability factors), but at this time can also conceptualize multiple emotions (compensatory factor) (Harter, 1984).

For every potentiating factor there may be a corresponding compensatory one. For example, if ambivalent attachment is a vulnerability factor, then a secure attachment is a protective factor (Cicchetti and Schneider-Rosen, in press). It is obvious then, that in listing compensatory and protective factors, their opposites may be assumed. Both members of a pair of opposites are included in Table 1 if they are of particular salience and importance.

The action of risk factors can differ. Some are mechanism-specific, whereas others operate in a general fashion. A factor is mechanism-specific if it potentiates or compensates by playing a role in a proposed mechanism of childhood depression, whereas its action is general if it can operate in a variety of ways in a variety of circumstances. For example, the loss of an ambivalently loved object is mechanism-specific, since it is a challenger according to the psychoanalytic theory of depression, whereas low socioeconomic status and nutritional deficiency operate in a general manner.

Our proposed model argues that we must examine all categories of risk factors and their transactions over time in order to understand the occurrence and specific form of childhood depression. While there are multiple etiologies for childhood depression, a vulnerable child, a vulnerable parent, environmental challenge, and a relative absence of compensatory protective factors and buffers may be involved in any combination. According to our model, childhood depression is expressed only when potentiating factors override compensatory ones, and some theoretical threshold is crossed. Anything reducing vulnerability and stress or increasing buffers or protective factors should decrease the probability of childhood depression.

This model is a framework within which one may account for the possibility of developing a depressive episode at any time. Implicit in the model is the assumption that the presence or absence of a depressive episode represents neither enduring nor transient influences alone, but rather a multiplicity of factors that need to be considered in combination with one another in order to account for and adequately explain the process whereby a specific depressive outcome has been achieved. We have illustrated the necessity of considering the transactions among child, caregiver, and environment in order to account adequately for current adaptation or maladaptation in children at risk for depression.

Since a transactional model of development is dynamic, time becomes an especially important dimension in its operation. Accordingly, as depicted in Figure 1, an initial early vulnerability to childhood depression can lead to several possible outcomes, including depression; however, the presence of a depressive episode — or some other risk factor — does not guarantee that depression will be the outcome found in subsequent assessments. Rather, various adaptations or maladaptations might result, with each possible outcome being multiply determined by the child, parent, environment transaction at the time of the assessment.

Conclusion

The basic tenets and principles of the organizational perspective provide the guiding assumptions for formulating research questions

Figure 1. Causal Relationships Between Vulnerability to Childhood Depression and Depressive Episodes, Later Maladaptation, or Later Adaptation

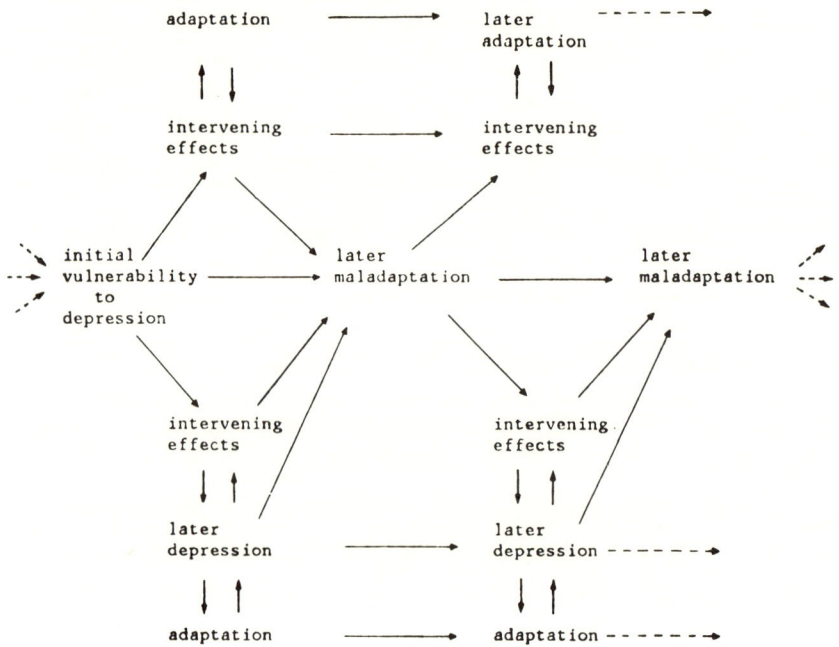

and for designing the appropriate empirical studies for testing theoretical propositions that concern coherence of development in both normal and clinical populations of children (Cicchetti and Pogge-Hesse, 1982; Cicchetti and Schneider-Rosen, in press). Researchers who adopt this perspective examine the ways in which behavior becomes hierarchically organized into more complex patterns within developmental systems, the manner in which later modes and functions evolve from earlier prototypes, and the processes by which global and diffuse part functions become integrated into wholes. This developmental approach emphasizes the relationships among cognitive, social, emotional, and neurophysiological systems, as well as the consequences of advances or lags within one system for the functioning of other systems. Moreover, an attempt is made to understand the effects of early experiences for later adaptation, while simultaneously considering the individual's current level of functioning and the influence of familial, social, and environmental factors.

We believe that greater progress will be made in unraveling the conundrum of childhood depression when this developmental approach is adopted. More specifically, it is our contention that this developmental perspective will provide information essential to the delineation of diagnostic criteria, to the understanding of etiology, course, and prognosis, for the assessment of competence or incompetence in the different behavioral domains, and for the application of therapeutic interventions that are congruent with the child's age and level of functioning. Throughout this chapter, we have stated that it is only when descriptive and theoretical formulations of depression take into account the biological reorganizations and the changing integration of competencies in the social, emotional, and cognitive domains that a more comprehensive understanding of childhood depression may be achieved and that methods for diagnosis and therapeutic intervention may be improved.

References

Ainsworth, M. D. S. "The Development of Infant-Mother Attachment." In B. Caldwell and H. Ricciuti (Eds.), *Review of Child Development.* Vol. III. Chicago: University of Chicago Press, 1973.

Akiskal, H. S., and McKinney, W. T., Jr. "Overview of Recent Research in Depression: Integration of Ten Conceptual Models into a Comprehensive Clinical Frame." *Archives of General Psychiatry,* 1975, *32,* 285–305.

American Psychiatric Association. *Diagnostic and Statistical Manual of Mental Disorders.* (3rd ed.) Washington, D. C.: Amerian Psychiatric Association, 1980.

Bischof, N. "A Systems Approach Toward the Functional Connections of Attachment and Fear." *Child Development,* 1975, *46,* 801–817.

Bowlby, J. *Attachment and Loss.* Vol. I: *Attachment.* New York: Basic Books, 1969.

Bowlby, J. *Attachment and Loss.* Vol. III. *Loss, Sadness, and Depression.* New York: Basic Books, 1980.

Carnap, R. "Testability and Meaning." *Philosphy of Science,* 1936, *3,* 420–471.

Cicchetti, D. "The Emergence of Developmental Psychopathology." *Child Development,* 1984, *55,* 1–7.

Cicchetti, D., and Pogge-Hesse, P. "Possible Contributions of the Study of Organically Retarded Persons to Developmental Theory." In E. Zigler and D. Balla (Eds.), *Mental Retardation: The Developmental-Difference Controversy.* Hillsdale, N.J.: Erlbaum, 1982.

Cicchetti, D., and Schneider-Rosen, K. "Theoretical and Empirical Considerations in the Investigation of the Relationship Between Affect and Cognition in Atypical Populations of Infants: Contributions to the Formulation of an Integrative Theory of Development." In C. Izard, J. Kagan, and R. Zajonc (Eds.), *Emotions, Cognition, and Behavior.* New York: Cambridge University Press, 1984.

Cicchetti, D., and Schneider-Rosen, K. "An Organizational Approach to Childhood Depression." In M. Rutter, C. Izard, and P. Read (Eds.), *Depression in Childhood: Developmental Perspectives.* New York: Guilford Press, in press.

Engel, G. "The Need for a New Medical Model: A Challenge for Biomedicine." *Science,* 1977, *196,* 129–135.

Gaensbauer, T. J. "Anaclitic Depression in a Three-and-One-Half-Month-Old Child." *American Journal of Psychiatry,* 1980, *137,* 841–842.

Gaensbauer, T. J., Harmon, R., Cytryn, L., and McKnew, D. H. "Social and Affective Development in Infants with a Manic-Depressive Parent." *American Journal of Psychiatry*, 1984, *141*, 223-229.

George, C. E., and Main, M. "Social Interactions of Young Abused Children: Approach, Avoidance, and Aggression." *Child Development*, 1979, *50*, 306-318.

Gottesman, I., and Shields, J. *Schizophrenia and Genetics: A Twin Study Vantage Point.* New York: Academic Press, 1972.

Harter, S. "Developmental Perspectives on the Self System." In P. Mussen (Ed.), *Handbook of Child Psychology.* New York: Wiley, 1984.

Kaplan, B. "The Study of Language in Psychiatry: The Comparative Developmental Approach and Its Application to Symbolization and Language in Psychopathology." In S. Arieti (Ed.), *American Handbook of Psychiatry.* Vol. 1. New York: Basic, 1966.

Kashani, J. H., Husain, A., Shekim, W. O., Hodges, K. K., Cytryn, L., and McKnew, D. H. "Current Perspectives on Childhood Depression: An Overview." *The American Journal of Psychiatry*, 1981, *138* (2), 143-153.

Meehl, P. E. "Schizotaxia, Schizotypy, Schizophrenia." *American Psychologist*, 1962, *17*, 827-838.

Meehl, P. E. "Specific Genetic Etiology, Psychodynamics, and Therapeutic Nihilism." *International Journal of Mental Health*, 1972, *1*, 10-27.

Meehl, P. E. "Theoretical Risks and Tabular Asterisks: Sir Karl, Sir Ronald, and the Slow Progress of Soft Psychology." *Journal of Consulting and Clinical Psychology*, 1978, *46* (4), 806-834.

Miller, J. *Living Systems.* New York: McGraw-Hill, 1978.

Pap, A. "Disposition Concepts and Extension Logic." In H. Feigl, M. Scriven, and G. Maxwell (Eds.), *Minnesota Studies in the Philosophy of Science.* Vol. II. Minneapolis: University of Minnesota Press, 1958.

Piaget, J. *The Origins of Intelligence.* New York: Norton, 1952.

Puig-Antich, J. "Affective Disorders in Childhood: A Review and Perspective." *Psychiatric Clinics of North America*, 1980, *3*, 403-424.

Puig-Antich, J., Chambers, W., Halpern, F., Hanlon, C., and Sachar, E. J. "Cortisol Hypersecretion in Prepubertal Depressive Illness." *Psychoneuroendocrinology*, 1979, *4*, 191-197.

Puig-Antich, J., and Gittelman, R. "Depression in Childhood and Adolescence." In E. S. Paykel (Ed.), *Handbook of Affective Disorders.* New York: Guilford, 1982.

Puig-Antich, J., Novacenko, H., Davies, M., Chambers, W. J., Tabrizi, M. A., Krawiec, V., Ambrosini, P. J., and Sachar, E. J. "Growth Hormone Secretion in Prepubertal Children with Major Depression." *Archives of General Psychiatry*, 1984, *41* (5), 455-460.

Puig-Antich, J., Perel, J. M., Lupartkin, W., Chambers, W. J., Shea, C., Tabrizi, M., and Stiller, R. L. "Plasma Levels of Imipramine (IMI) and Desmethylimipramine (DMI) and Clinical Response to Prepubertal Major Depressive Disorder." *Journal of American Academy of Child Psychiatry*, 1979, *18*, 616-627.

Rie, H. E. "Depression in Childhood: A Survey of Some Pertinent Contributions." *Journal of the American Academy of Child Psychiatry*, 1966, *5*, 653-685.

Rutter, M. "The Developmental Psychopathology of Depression: Issues and Perspectives." In M. Rutter, C. Izard, and P. Read (Eds.), *Depression in Childhood: Developmental Perspectives.* New York: Guilford, in press.

Sameroff, A., and Chandler, M. "Reproductive Risk and the Continuum of Caretaking Casualty." In F. Horowitz (Ed.), *Review of Child Development Research.* Vol. 4. Chicago: University of Chicago Press, 1975.

Sandler, J., and Joffe, W. G. "Notes on Childhood Depression." *International Journal of Psychoanalysis*, 1965, *46*, 88-96.

Schneider-Rosen, K., Braunwald, K., Carlson, V., and Cicchetti, D. "Current Perspectives in Attachment Theory: Illustration from the Study of Maltreated Infants." In I. Bretherton and E. Waters (Eds.), *Growing Points in Attachment Theory and Research. Monographs of the Society for Research in Child Development,* in press.

Sellars, W. S. "Counterfactuals, Dispositions, and the Causal Modalities." In H. Fiegl, M. Scriven, and G. Maxwell (Eds.), *Minnesota Studies in the Philosophy of Science.* Vol. II. Minneapolis: University of Minnesota Press, 1958.

Spitzer, R. L., Endicott, J., and Robins, E. "Research Diagnostic Criteria: Rationale and Reliability." *Archives of General Psychiatry,* 1978, *35,* 773–782.

Sroufe, L. A. "The Coherence of Individual Development." *American Psychologist,* 1979, *34,* 834–841.

Sroufe, L. A., and Rutter, M. "The Domain of Developmental Psychopathology." *Child Development,* 1984, *55,* 17–29.

Sylvester, C. E., Burke, P. M., McCauley, E. A., and Clark, C. J. "Manic Psychosis in Childhood: Report of Two Cases." *The Journal of Nervous and Mental Disease,* 1984, *172* (1), 12–15.

Von Bertalanffy, L. *General Systems Theory: Foundations, Development, Applications.* New York: Braziller, 1968.

Waddington, C. H. *Principles of Development and Differentiation.* New York: Macmillan, 1966.

Waters, E., and Sroufe, L. A. "Competence as a Developmental Construct." *Developmental Review,* 1983, *3,* 79–97.

Werner, H. *Comparative Psychology of Mental Development.* New York: International Universities Press, 1948.

Werner, H., and Kaplan, B. *Symbol Formation: An Organismic-Developmental Approach to Language and the Expression of Thought.* New York: Wiley, 1963.

Zahn-Waxler, C., Cummings, E. M., McKnew, D., and Radke-Yarrow, M. "Altruism, Aggression and Social Interactions in Young Children with a Manic-Depressive Parent." *Child Development,* 1984, *55,* 112–122.

Zahn-Waxler, C., McKnew, D. H., Cummings, E. M., Davenport, Y. B., and Radke-Yarrow, M. "Problem Behaviors and Peer Interactions of Young Children with a Manic-Depressive Parent." *The American Journal of Psychiatry,* 1984, *141* (2), 236–240.

Zubin, J., and Spring, B. "Vulnerability: A New View of Schizophrenia." *Journal of Abnormal Psychology,* 1977, *56,* 103–126.

Dante Cicchetti is the Norman Tishman Associate Professor of Psychology and Social Relations at Harvard University. His research interests lie in the areas of developmental psychopathology, affective disorders, child maltreatment, socio-emotional development, and the neurosciences.

Karen Schneider-Rosen is an assistant professor in the Department of Psychology at Boston College. Her research interests lie in the areas of developmental psychopathology, childhood depression, child maltreatment, and social and emotional development.

An important early step in the classification of childhood depression from a developmental perspective is the identification of age-specific signs and symptoms. Assessment must take into account the child's level of functioning within the cognitive, social, and affective domains.

The Developmental Progression of Depression in Female Children

Judy Garber

In a relatively brief period of time, childhood depression has gone from being essentially overlooked (for example, Kanner, 1957), to having its existence challenged and denied (Mahler, 1961; Rie, 1966; Rochlin, 1959), to being accepted as a distinct entity whose defining characteristics are isomorphic with its adult counterpart (Cytryn and others, 1980). Although there were some early case studies reported in the literature (Anthony, 1977; Saussure, 1947), it really was not until the

---

This research was supported in part by a National Research Service Award from the National Institute of Mental Health, 1F31, MH08493-01 and a Dissertation Fellowship from the University of Minnesota.

I would like to express my extreme gratitude to the staff at Washburn Child Guidance Clinic and at the Psychological Services of the Minneapolis Public School System for allowing me the opportunity to conduct my research at their facilities and for their continued support and cooperation.

I would also like to thank the members of my dissertation committee for their encouragement including Paul Meehl, adviser, Norman Garmezy, Alan Sroufe, Auke Tellegen, and Carl Malmquist. Finally, sincere thanks to Mary Jones for her secretarial assistance in preparing the manuscript.

journal *The Nervous Child* (1952) devoted a special issue to manic-depressive illness in childhood that depression among elementary-school-age children received any attention. The discussions that followed in the subsequent decade were concerned with whether in fact depression in childhood was psychodynamically possible, and if it really did exist. The predominant view at the time among psychoanalytic theorists was that depressive disorders could not occur in children because children lack a well-internalized superego before adolescence (Rie, 1966; Rochlin, 1959), and because "the ego cannot sustain itself without taking prompt defensive actions against object loss. It cannot survive in an objectless state for any length of time" (Mahler, 1961, p. 339).

A related perspective held during the same time was that depression in children is "masked," that is, expressed in behavioral equivalent; it could not be directly observed. Proponents of this view (Glaser, 1967; Toolan, 1962) suggested that children do not manifest the signs and symptoms of adult depressive reaction, but rather manifest symptoms of other disorders instead, such as conduct disorders, separation anxiety, enuresis, and somatic complaints. Glaser (1967) argued that although the child does not present symptoms that are typically associated with depression, the child's psychopathology features depressive elements that are dynamic forces influencing the child's functioning.

Critics of the concept of masked depression have emphasized the fact that the various disorders that have been characterized as masking depression include practically the full range of possible psychopathological disorders of childhood (Gittelman-Klein, 1977; Kovacs and Beck, 1977). Moreover, the connection between these various disorders and the presumed underlying depressive feature is unclear. No criteria have been given for how to tell when a disorder is masking depression and when it can be taken at face value.

The trend in the last decade has been to accept the existence of childhood depression as a real clinical phenomenon, and to search for its defining characteristics. Early attempts to build a set of diagnostic criteria started from the viewpoint that childhood depressive disorder has a number of similarities to the adult syndrome as well as having some additional unique features specific to children (Brumback and others, 1977; Weinberg and others, 1973). Proponents of this viewpoint maintain that childhood depression includes symptoms similar to the adult disorder—sadness, low self-esteem, loss of energy, sleep problems, and eating disturbance—as well as other symptoms that are not typically part of the adult syndrome—social withdrawal, somatic complaints, and aggression.

At least a dozen different sets of criteria have been suggested and used in the various studies in the literature. Because of the lack of a standardized, agreed-upon set of diagnostic criteria for defining childhood depression, several investigators (Cytryn and others, 1980; Puig-Antich and others, 1978) recently have recommended the universal acceptance and use of DSM-III criteria for major affective disorders in adults to establish the same diagnosis for children. Although this has the potential advantage of providing uniformity across researchers, empirical research is needed to determine whether these criteria are in fact valid for use with children. Thus, it seems that in a very brief period of time the field has gone from the one extreme of denying the very existence of depression in children to the other of asserting that depressive disorders in children and adults are isomorphic.

Recently, this latter perspective—that the childhood and adult forms of depressive disorder are isomorphic—has been challenged by developmental psychopathologists (Cicchetti and Schneider-Rosen, in press; Sroufe and Rutter, 1984). These writers assert that from a developmental perspective it is unrealistic to expect behavioral isomorphism in observed signs or symptoms of depression in children of different ages because there are important differences in the developmental progression of children's cognitive, linguistic, and socioemotional capacities that will produce differences in their interpretation, experience, and expression of depressive symptomatology over time. Therefore, the search for appropriate diagnostic criteria must incorporate age-specific manifestations of the symptomatology as well as broader notions of adaptation and competence.

The lack of a well-articulated and reliable set of criteria for diagnosing depression in children has been a major obstacle to progress in research in this field. In the absence of clear and objective guidelines for identifying depressive disorders in children, generalizations across studies and communicating among researchers has been difficult. A major prerequisite to the advancement of knowledge concerning childhood depression is the construction of a valid set of diagnostic criteria. It is essential that these diagnostic criteria be formulated and validated within a developmental framework.

The major goal of the present paper is to examine the depressive syndrome and the symptoms that comprise it from a developmental perspective. First, the developmental perspective will be described and its implications for the diagnosis and classification of childhood depression will be discussed. Theoretical and empirical literature that has specifically attempted to approach the problem of the classification of childhood depression within a developmental framework will be reviewed.

Then, results of a research project designed to address the question of the developmental progression of depressive symptomatology will be presented. Finally, the implications of these findings for a developmentally oriented classification and diagnosis of depression will be proposed.

The Developmental Perspective

Recently, there have been several attempts to define a developmental perspective for the domain of childhood psychopathology in general (Sroufe and Rutter, 1984) and for childhood depression in particular (Cicchetti and Schneider-Rosen, in press). Garber (1984) has outlined the implications of such a developmental perspective for the classification of childhood disorders. The central focus of the developmental perspective of psychopathology is on the continuities and discontinuities between normality and disorder and between one developmental period and the next.

The three axioms of the developmental perspective are derived from basic developmental theory:

1. The progression of development is described best by the orthogenetic principle (Werner, 1948), which states that development proceeds from a state of relative globality and lack of differentiation to a state of increasing complexity, integration, and hierarchic organization. Despite periods of reorganization and transformation of overt behavior, however, the individual's coherence is maintained through hierarchic integration of the individual's early structures (Cicchetti and Schneider-Rosen, in press).
2. Development is a series of behavioral reorganizations around specific salient developmental issues. The quality of the individual's adaptation, or the "fit" between the child and his or her environment, may be judged with respect to how well the child negotiates the salient issues for the particular developmental period (Matas and others, 1978; Sroufe and Rutter, 1984).
3. Developmental issues are broadly integrative and cut across affective, social, and cognitive domains. The individual's current level of functioning is assessed in terms of the level of adaptation in each of these domains. Moreover, the developmental approach is concerned with the interrelationships between the cognitive, emotional, and social systems, particularly with respect to how advances or lags within one sys-

tem may affect the functioning of other systems (Cicchetti and Pogge-Hesse, 1982).

These three aspects of basic development theory are fundamental to understanding psychopathology within a developmental framework. According to developmentalists, psychopathology results from "the lack of organization or integration of social, emotional, or cognitive competences that may influence the successful resolution or completion of the salient developmental tasks that need to be accomplished in each domain" (Cicchetti and Schneider-Rosen, in press, p. 13). Maladaptation is defined in terms of incompetence or deviation in the completion of developmentally-defined tasks (Sroufe, 1979) or in terms of failure to deal with phase-appropriate experiences (Greenspan and others, 1979). Thus, it is necessary to have an adequate knowledge of normal development in the various affective, cognitive, and social domains in order to recognize deviations from age-appropriate expectations.

The developmental perspective on psychopathology focuses on at least three fundamental issues:

1. *Prediction.* It is important to determine the link between earlier adaptation and later pathology (Sroufe and Rutter, 1984). The developmental perspective allows us to examine individual coherence with respect to both failures in adaptation as well as nonpathological patterns that predict later pathology.

2. *Origin and time course disorders.* The origins of adult psychopathology may not be in childhood disorders of a similar type; the antecedents of pathology may be found in early failures in adaptation to developmental tasks.

3. *Behavioral manifestations.* Developmental psychopathologists assume that manifestations of disorders vary with development as a result of changing capacities in the growing child. Developmental advances within each of the behavioral domains (affective, cognitive, and social) are likely to influence the expression and meaning of a behavior (Cicchetti and Schneider-Rosen, in press).

It is interesting that the three issues of psychopathology emphasized by the developmental perspective roughly correspond to three elements of traditional psychiatric nosology—prognosis, etiology, and clinical symptomatology, respectively. It is clear, however, that the developmental perspective dictates that a somewhat new approach be taken to the problem of the classification of childhood psychopathology. Despite arguments to the contrary (Santostefano, 1971), the developmental model is not by definition antagonistic to nosology. Rather, the developmental perspective complements the standard diagnostic classification schema (Greenspan and others, 1979) by highlighting new dimensions, variables, and parameters that need to be incorporated into a more inclusive and extensive nosology.

According to Garber (1984), the central issues in the classification of childhood psychopathology are the continuity between childhood and adult psychopathology, and the definition and classification of normality and adaptation. The study of continuity raises subsidiary issues: The diagnostic criteria that define adult psychopathology, if left unmodified, may be inappropriate for use with children. Maturational differences influence children's abilities to experience or express certain affects, cognitions, and behaviors. Thus, the manner in which an individual expresses symptoms may vary over the course of development. The validity of a diagnosis during childhood is not necessarily dependent on there being future episodes of the disorder over the course of development into adulthood. Moreover, adult psychopathology need not be preceded by a similar disorder during childhood. The natural course and prognosis of a childhood disorder should be assessed independently of its continuity with adult psychopathology. Finally, the continuity between childhood and adult psychopathology may be reflected more accurately in terms of patterns of adaptation than in terms of behavioral isomorphism of discrete symptoms across time.

The second implication of the developmental perspective is that we must understand normal development in the affective, cognitive, and social domains in order to recognize and assess deviation from expected patterns at each age level. A classification of psychopathology that meshes with some notion of what is the normal progression of development in each of these various domains will help the assessment of a child's current level of functioning and of the child's progress over time, relative to an expected baseline. This system of classification will enable us to identify the type of impaired functioning associated with particular disorders, as well as to examine the impact of advances or lags in one domain on another domain within both normal and atypical populations.

Finally, the developmental perspective highlights the need for broadening the content of current classification systems beyond symptom description. Because development takes place in the context of phase-specific developmental tasks, and adaptation and maladaptation are judged with respect to the successful or unsuccessful negotiation of these tasks, classification systems of developmental psychopathology should include a systematic categorization of levels of adaptation to the various developmental tasks. The classification scheme used in the assessment of the quality of infant-mother relationships (Ainsworth and others, 1978), and the developmental structuralist approach to classification proposed by Greenspan and others (1979) are good examples of preliminary efforts to categorize patterns of adaptation to such developmental tasks as attachment, homeostasis, and internalization. Thus, the developmental perspective highlights the need for reexamining traditional notions of classification and expanding our current systems to go beyond symptom description.

The Developmental Perspective on Childhood Depression. What are the implications of the developmental perspective for the classification of childhood depression in particular? The major issue for research in the area of childhood depression has been finding the appropriate diagnostic criteria for identifying the disorder in children. Although historically the tendency was to deny the existence of the syndrome in children or to assert that it only could be recognized in masked forms, the current trend is to apply the adult criteria, essentially unmodified, to children.

Developmental psychopathologists, however, have begun to question this current trend, and argue that the adult-based diagnostic criteria do not take sufficient account of possible age-related differences in the defining attributes or in the manifest expression of the syndrome (Kovacs, in press). Cicchetti and Schneider-Rosen (in press) suggest further that we would not expect to find behavioral isomorphism in observed signs or symptoms of depression in children of different ages, and therefore it is futile to try to define by symptom characteristics a diagnostic picture for depression that can be applied across ages. Developmental advances in cognitive structures and functions especially influence the manner in which children experience, interpret, and express emotions at different ages.

An alternative, and somewhat less pessimistic view of the diagnostic enterprise is that the search for symptomatic isomorphism is not futile, but is insufficient. Using the developmental perspective as a guide, it may be possible to identify age-appropriate signs and symptoms that take into consideration the child's level of functioning within the various cognitive, affective, and social domains. The developmental perspective does not dictate that we abandon symptom-complex diagnosis, but rather that we go beyond it by (1) identifying additional phase-specific manifestations of the syndrome while eliminating other age-inappropriate symptoms, (2) broadening the existing definitions of symptoms to encompass developmental differences in phenomenology, and (3) widening the focus beyond symptoms to include new categories of functioning such as levels of adaptation and competence. Empirical investigations may reveal that certain symptoms of the adult depressive syndrome are not appropriate for use with children and should be eliminated from the syndrome definition. Such symptoms as guilt and hopelessness that require a higher level of cognitive functioning are potential examples of this. On the other hand, there may be other symptoms not typically associated with the adult syndrome that are found to cluster about the childhood syndrome and, therefore, should be added to it. Aggression and somatic complaints, for example, may reflect children's less mature coping strategies and defensive style.

Once the salient developmental issues for the various age levels are identified and the modes of adaptation and maladaptation to them are categorized, these patterns of adaptation can be incorporated into the diagnostic process. Learning to cope with loss, developing a sense of self, and establishing adequate social relationships all probably have the potential to affect the development and maintenance of childhood depression. Therefore clinicians and researchers must examine these spheres in addition to the specific discrete symptomatology.

Finally, the developmental perspective has implications for both the operational definitions used to describe the symptoms and the methods used to assess them. It may be that the general areas of dysfunction associated with depression, such as affective, cognitive, vegetative, and behavioral areas, are similar across development, but the specific symptoms and behaviors that characterize dysfunction vary with age. Therefore, the definition of the symptom or area of dysfunction should be broad enough to include age-appropriate manifestations. A simple example is anhedonia: In adults this symptom typically is assessed in terms of loss of interest in sex or usual hobbies; for children, it is more appropriately defined in terms of sustained periods of boredom and loss of interest in usually pleasurable activities. The affective component of depression is a somewhat more complex example. Depressed adults typically describe the predominant affect that they feel to be sadness. Children, however, particularly young ones, are less likely to directly verbalize a feeling of sadness. Rather, they may simply appear to be sad and tearful or they may use different words to describe their feelings — for example, "rotten," "lousy," or "bad." Before accepting any of these words as synonyms for "sad" — or, at least as related terms — we need to conduct normative developmental studies of children's expression of affect to see if we are observing an age-appropriate behavior. We can further check the validity of broad age-appropriate definitions of symptoms by collecting data to see whether these symptoms cluster in a meaningful syndrome with a particular etiology, course, prognosis, and response to treatment.

In sum, early steps in the classification of childhood depression from a developmental perspective are: (1) determine whether the expression of depressive symptoms varies with development, (2) identify additional age-appropriate symptoms and areas of dysfunction to include in the diagnostic process, and (3) assess the influence of children's cognitive, affective, and social competencies and their physiological maturation on the experience and the expression of depressive symptoms. To date there has been only limited theoretical work and even fewer empirical investigations of childhood depression from a developmental perspective. Study has focused primarily on different symptom manifestations of depression with age. The remainder of the article will provide a brief review of this literature and then will present a recent investigation designed to expand this work by addressing the question of the differential symptom picture of childhood depression at different ages.

Developmental Approaches to the Classification of Childhood Depression

Specific developmental approaches to the classification of childhood depression have been, for the most part, anecdotal or theoretical (for example, Bemporad and Wilson, 1978; Glaser, 1967; Malmquist, 1971). In general, these conceptual attempts to examine childhood depression developmentally have tended to divide children into the four broad age categories of infancy, preschool, school age, and adolescence. The focus of this literature has been on the issue of the existence of the disorder at the different ages, and the similarities and differences in its phenomenology over the course of development.

Infancy. There are several syndromes that have been identified in infants as being analogous symptomatically to adult depression, including anaclitic depression (Spitz, 1946), conservation-withdrawal reaction (Engel and Reichsman, 1956), and failure to thrive. Spitz (1946) described *anaclitic depression* as a reaction to separation from the mother that is characterized by three phases: protest, rejection, and, finally, withdrawal. The symptoms that are most noteworthy because of the similarity to adult depression include: listlessness, apathy, minimal movement, loss of weight, sleep disturbance, crying, unresponsiveness, and marked withdrawal. Not surprisingly, cognitive symptoms of depression, such as low self-esteem, guilt, and hopelessness, are not seen in infants because infants do not yet have any awareness of self, nor do they have any representational thought until approximately eighteen months (Piaget, 1954). There is considerable debate as to whether these early syndromes have any relevance to or continuity with childhood or adult forms of the disorder (Bemporad and Wilson, 1978). This debate is a good example of the problem of whether similar symptoms and behaviors mean the same thing at different ages. Sandler and Joffe (1965) prefer to describe the clinical picture that Spitz calls anaclitic depression as a "basic psychobiological reaction to deprivation." In support of this idea, Bemporad and Wilson (1978) point out that infants may display a syndrome similar to the maternal deprivation syndrome when faced with a lack of cognitive stimulation, nutritional deficiency, or organic deficiency diseases. Moreover, Engle and Reichsman (1956) suggested that there is a basic biological pattern known as *conservation-withdrawal* that serves as an instinctive prototype of later depression although they do not equate the reaction during infancy with depression itself. Thus, depression in infancy remains a questionable phenomenon. There appears to be a syndrome that resembles the adult disorder with respect to many of its vegetative and behavioral symptoms. The continuity of this syndrome with that found in older children and adults, however, remains to be determined. Finally, the infant syndrome does seem to indicate that early deprivation and the formation of adequate attachments may be potentially salient issues in the development of depression.

Preschool Children. The existence and manifestations of depressive syndromes in preschool children also are controversial. Depressive symptoms observed in this age group include brief periods of sadness, weepiness, loss of interest in activities, feeling rejected, physical complaints, temper tantrums, and aggression (Commins and Heisler, 1980). It is rare, however, to see a cluster of these symptoms appearing in the same child for a sustained period of time. Rather, these symptoms are more typically seen as transient reactions to an immediate stressor.

There is a paucity of clinical reports of children of this age who manifest the full syndrome. Poznanski and Zrull (1970), after reviewing a large set of records from the outpatient department of a children's hospital, found only one child under the age of five who appeared to display depressive symptoms. Brumback and Weinberg (1979) have presented case histories of episodes of depression and mania in preschoolers. From the material presented, however, it is difficult to separate descriptions of temperament and episodic but normal developmental regressions from more serious psychopathology.

In a review of one hundred children who had had at least one episode of depression, Ushakov and Girich (1972) reported that the clinical picture for twelve children under seven years old whom they observed was diffuse and symptomatically undefined. These children did appear to be sad, wept frequently, were sluggish in their movements, and showed decreased interest in play activities although it was relatively easy to divert them. Psychomotor symptoms were the least stable, with a tendency to find an increase in restlessness and fidgety behavior toward evening. Notably absent were suicide attempts, delusions, and verbal complaints of melancholy.

Bemporad and Wilson (1978) attribute the fairly transient nature of depressive symptoms in young children largely to their tendency to live for the moment, their inability to generalize from one experience to another, and their limited sense of past and future. The cognitive and affectual limitations of the preoperational period suggest that the manifestation of depressive symptomatology may differ for this age group, and that it may be necessary to conceptualize the syndrome somewhat differently and to use alternative strategies for assessing its presence in these children. Again, the relationship of symptoms resembling depression to later disorder is unclear, although Bemporad and Wilson (1978) suggest that the children who present with a serious, inhibited, clingy depressive picture are, at least, at risk for future psychopathology, particularly of a depressive nature.

School-Aged Children. Depression in school-aged children has been more extensively studied and tends to be more common than in the younger age groups. For a long time, however, both in the clinic and in research, depression was overshadowed by the more predominant disorders characteristic of this age period—conduct disorders and emotional disorders. Most of the writing dealing with masked depression refer to school-aged children.

Because children undergo important developmental changes during the school-age years (ages six to twelve), there has been a tendency not to lump this age group together in phenomenologic studies of depression. Bemporad and Wilson (1978) divide the period roughly into middle and late childhood and suggest that in middle childhood there are longer periods of sadness than found in younger children, although this sadness is still primarily seen in overt, rather than verbal, behavior. Children in middle childhood also still lack the cognitive capacity to sustain a low self-esteem. Finally, their sadness still tends to be a reaction to an external situation, and is typically quite appropriate to the reality of the situation, as contrasted with the distorted thinking reportedly observed among some adult depressives (Beck, 1967). During late childhood, children's increasingly complex and differentiated cognitive apparatus has developed to a point where they can think logically as well as begin to distort reality (Flavell, 1977). Children's developing perspective-taking ability allows them to infer motives and attribute beliefs to others. They can also begin to perceive intentionality in their own and others' actions, as well as to misattribute blame, thereby opening themselves up to the experience of self-blame and guilt. A very significant change during this period is the development of a more stable sense of self (Damon and Hart, 1982). This allows children in late childhood to make judgments about themselves — to compare themselves with their peers and their ego ideal — that could result in negative, self-derogatory conclusions often associated with depression. Thus, by late childhood, cognitive structures have developed to a point that the child can experience many of the depressive symptoms that require active mental interpretations rather than passive responses to the environment (Bemporad and Wilson, 1978).

There is some limited empirical work supporting the notion of variation in depressive phenomenology with development. In contrasting children in the seven- to ten-year old age groups ($n = 24$) with children under seven, Ushakov and Girich (1972) found the following symptomology for the older group: (1) Depressive symptoms were more persistent; (2) the feelings of sadness were recognized and expressed by children, rather than simply observed in their behaviors; (3) symptoms of anxiety were found considerably less often than among younger children who experienced increased anxiety at night; (4) suicidal ideation was noted, although it tended to be associated with spiting others rather than self-reproach. The same study on depressive disturbances included young adolescents. In the eleven to thirteen-year-old group ($n = 26$), depressive symptoms were more fully expressed and pronounced. These children showed an even greater awareness of their illness and its cause than the late childhood group, and a further decrease in anxiety and behavioral disturbances. Rudimentary depressive delusional remarks were observed for the first time among some of these children. Thus, the advancing age through the school-age years and the characteristics of disorder apparent at younger ages seem to become more concrete and recognizable as symptoms typically associated with depression.

A second study to examine the differential manifestation of depressive symptoms across ages six through thirteen was conducted by McConville and others (1973). Reviewing the records of seventy-five inpatient children who had been described as being depressed, McConville and his colleagues (1973) selected fifteen depressive items on the basis of clinical frequency to be rated on a three-point scale for each child. They found that three age groups of children could be differentiated on the basis of their symptom pictures. Symptoms in the six to eight-year-old group were primarily of the "affectual type," that is, consisting of feelings of sadness, helplessness, loneliness, loss, and an unspecifid feeling of being bad. The second group, ages eight to ten years, were characterized by feelings of inability to help others, of being disliked, of hopelessness, and of negative self-esteem. This set of depressive symptoms was labeled the "self-esteem type." McConville and others (1973) suggested that the second group of children's more advanced abilities to openly verbalize their feelings and thoughts may have accounted for the shift toward more cognitive symptoms. The third type, seen in a subset of the ten to thirteen-year-olds was referred to as the "guilt type" of depression and included feelings of being wicked or hated, the belief that one was being justly punished, and suicidal ideation. The intensity of these self-attacking thoughts of wickedness, however, was notably less than is found in adult depressive psychoses.

In sum, these empirical findings provide support for the existence of differences in depressive symptomatology with age that appear to be meaningful developmentally. There appears to be a trend toward decreasing diffuseness of the symptom picture and increasing similarity to the adult syndrome with the growing complexity and differentiation of cognitive, linguistic, affective, and social capacities.

Adolescence. When depression occurs during adolescence, it typically is characterized by symptoms similar to adult depression. These may include loss of interest, dysphoria, impaired concentration, fatigue, anorexia and overeating, feelings of worthlessness, and suicidal ideation (Carlson and Strober, 1979). Social withdrawal and hypochondriasis are also common. Carlson and Strober (1979) also note that classic endogenous symptoms (for example, loss of pleasure, guilt, psychomotor disturbance, sleep difficulties) are not uncommon in adolescents. They conclude that the unambiguous expression of depressive phenomenology is by no means rare before late adolescence.

Similarly, Ushakov and Girich (1972) found that among fourteen- to seventeen-year-old patients ($n = 20$), about one-third of the depressions differed little from those seen in adults. They observed genuine melancholy, motor and intellectual inhibition, and a significant rate of suicidal ideation and suicide attempts. Weepiness and mononeurotic symptoms were noticeably less frequent among adolescents than in the younger age groups.

Despite the increasing similarity to adult depression, however, depression in adolescence still presents some diagnostic difficulty. This is true in part because adolescent depression is often accompanied by serious behavior disorders such as delinquency, truancy, chemical abuse, and sexual promiscuity. Thus, as described earlier for younger children, the depressive symptoms may be overshadowed by more obvious behavioral aberrations. Diagnosis can also be impeded because a great deal of emotional turmoil, reflected in considerable lability of mood, characterize the period of adolescence. Significant physiological changes, peer pressure for approval, and societal demands for adult behavior make this a difficult time for even the most psychologically healthy young person. Normal mood fluctuations and variability in adaptation to these tasks are sometimes difficult to distinguish from a pathological response, making diagnosis of a disorder more complex. The diagnosis of depression in adolescence, therefore, is as much dependent on the duration, combination, and severity of the symptoms, as it is on the presence of the symptoms themselves.

This brief review has highlighted the developmental progression of depression in children. Sadness and several of the other depressive symptoms tend to be diffuse and less well-differentiated among young children. Adult depressive symptoms of self-blame, psychomotor retardation, hopelessness, and suicidal ideation only begin to emerge in late childhood, and do not become fully evident until adolescence. There also tends to be some decrease in crying and overactivity with age.

Considerable controversy remains regarding the meaning of these age differences. Do we conclude from the evidence that depressive disorder is simply uncommon in young children, or rather that the depression is expressed in a different form over the course of development (Rutter, 1980)? Examining the developmental progression of depressive phenomenology in the context of an understanding of normal development allows us to make predictions about what symptoms are likely to emerge at which point in development and to explain the reasons for these developmental transitions. From the developmental perspective, it becomes clear that there are cognitive, linguistic, and socioemotional competencies that develop at different rates and, hence, significantly influence the experience and expression of depressive symptomatology. Therefore, it seems reasonable to expect that certain symptoms of adult depression will be uncommon among young children, but that there may be age-appropriate manifestations of the broad areas of dysfunction that comprise a depression-like syndrome in children.

The literature reviewed in this chapter is predominantly theoretical and anecdotal. Only two empirical studies of the developmental progression of depression were noted (McConville and others, 1973; Ushakov and Girich, 1972). When these studies were conducted, neither well-defined operational criteria nor standardized assessment methods were in use. The project described in the following section used the most reliable criteria and assessment instruments currently available to address the question of whether the manner of expression of depressive symptomatology alters with development.

An Empirical Study

Method

Subjects. Subjects were 137 girls between the ages of seven and thirteen inclusive. The study was limited to one sex so that possible important differences in the pattern and clustering of behavior problems as a function of the sex of the child (Achenbach, 1978) would not confuse the results. Using the same criteria and categories of dysfunction for both sexes may not do justice to potential differences in their development. Females were chosen because (1) the ratio of females to males in nonbipolar affective disorders in adults tends to be approximately two to one (Weissman and Myers, 1978); (2) internalizers (for example, obsessive-compulsive, depressed) tend to outnumber externalizers (hyperactive, aggressive) about two to one among girls (Achenbach, 1966); and (3) emotional disorders were found to be somewhat more common among girls than boys (26:17) in the Isle of Wight project (Rutter and others, 1970). This particular age range was chosen because it encompasses significant changes in cognitive status and physical development. An upper range of thirteen years old was designated in order to keep the primary focus on prepubertal functioning, and a lower range of seven years was chosen because a certain level of cognitive development was required in order to complete the various questionnaires and tasks.

To be included in the study, children were required to show a full-scale Wechsler Intelligence Scale for Children–Revised (WISC-R) IQ of 70 or above. The mean IQ for the sample was 98.3 with a range of 70 to 135. The sample was predominantly Caucasian (79 percent).

Forty-five percent of the children's parents were married or remarried; 42 percent were divorced or separated. The majority of the children were living with a biological parent (88 percent); 9 percent were adopted.

Participating children were recruited consecutively from two different agencies. The first setting was a community child guidance clinic; the second source was the psychological services of the Minneapolis school system. The majority of the children using the child guidance clinic attended the same Minneapolis schools from which the second sample was obtained. Eighty-nine children were seen in the clinic; the remaining forty-eight children were referred from the schools. Both agencies dealt with various educational, emotional, and behavioral concerns. Approximately 25 percent of the combined sample had been referred for educational evaluations only. The remaining referrals had been made for a combination of reasons.

Procedure. Once a child was identified as being within the appropriate age range, parents were contacted by letter requesting their participation in the project. Children for whom permission was obtained were then entered into the study. All children were seen individually for at least two sessions; most were seen for three. The average sessions lasted for approximately ninety minutes. The full assessment typically took place over two weeks.

Assessment. The assessment battery involved a structured clinical interview of the child, and several questionnaires which were completed by the children, parents, teachers, and clinician. Only a subset of these measures will be described here.

Children's Depression Inventory (CDI). The CDI is a twenty-seven-item clinical research instrument suitable for use with children ages seven to thirteen (Kovacs, 1981). The items are presented in a three-choice format ranging from 0 to 2 in the direction of increasing severity, and cover an array of depressive symptoms. CDI total scores range from 0 to 54, with higher scores reflecting more severe depression. Because of concerns about illiteracy, all children were read the CDI.

Parent Form of the Children's Depression Inventory (P-CDI). The P-CDI was developed by Garber (1983) as a measure of children's depression to be completed by parents. The questionnaire is essentially identical to the CDI except that questions are worded so that parents respond according to how they believe their child feels, and not how they themselves feel regarding the item. Thus, the first twenty-seven items of the P-CDI are simply rewordings of the CDI, and yield a total score ranging from 0 to 54. An additional eight items are included at the end of the scale that ask parents to respond with their own feelings.

Children's Depression Rating Scale (CDRS). The CDRS was developed by Poznanski and others (1979) as a clinician's rating scale of depression. It is modeled after the Hamilton Depression Rating Scale for adults (Hamilton, 1969). The CDRS has undergone several revisions, and currently contains seventeen items, fourteen of which are rated along a continuum of severity from 0 to 7. The remaining three items are rated from 0 to 5. Thus, possible scores on the CDRS range from 0 to 113.

Poznanski and others (1979) recommend that the clinician's ratings on the CDRS be based on all available sources of information including the children, parents, teachers, and records. In the present study, the CDRS ratings were based on (1) an interview with the children based on the Schedule for Affective Disorders and Schizophrenia for school-aged children (Kiddie-SADS) developed by Puig-Antich and Chambers (1979), and the Diagnostic Interview for Children and Adolescents (DICA) (Herjanic and others, 1975); (2) a review of specific depression-relevant items from an expanded (273-item) version of the Child Behavior Checklist (Achenbach and Edelbrock, 1979) completed by both parents and teachers; and (3) school and medical records.

In the present study, the CDRS ratings were made without use of knowledge of scores on the CDI and P-CDI. This blind assessment later enabled us to assess the concurrent validity of the CDI and the P-CDI in relation to an independent criteria (CDRS).

Results

Demographic Data. There were no significant differences on the basis of either age or depression for race, IQ, reason for referral, or referral agency. There was a significant relationship between age and parental marital status $[F(2,134) = 4.69, p < .01]$, and age and family status $[F(2,134) = 6.76, p < .01]$, indicating that the older children were more likely to have parents who were not currently married, and that more older than younger children were living with someone other than a biological parent. A significant relationship also was found between depression and parental marital status $[F(1,135) = 5.18, p < .05]$, indicating that the depressed children were more likely to have parents who were not currently married.

Comparison of Syndrome Depression as a Function of Age. Children were divided into depressed versus nondepressed according to whether or not they met the criteria for the syndrome of depression as defined in DSM-III. In the present analyses, no distinction was made between primary and secondary depression (Robins and Guze, 1969). Children in the depressed group manifest a syndrome of depression, but may not necessarily be diagnosed as having Major Affective Disorder.

In the present sample, 64 children (47 percent) met criteria for syndrome depression, but half of these children ($n = 32$) had other syndromes as well, particularly anxiety and separation anxiety as well as conduct disorder, attention deficit disorder, and enuresis. Figure 1 shows the percent of children at each age who manifested syndrome depression. It is noteworthy that the rate of depression increases markedly for the oldest group (ages twelve to thirteen).

In all of the remaining analyses children were grouped accord-

Figure 1. Percent of Children at Each Age Who Met Criteria for Syndrome Depression

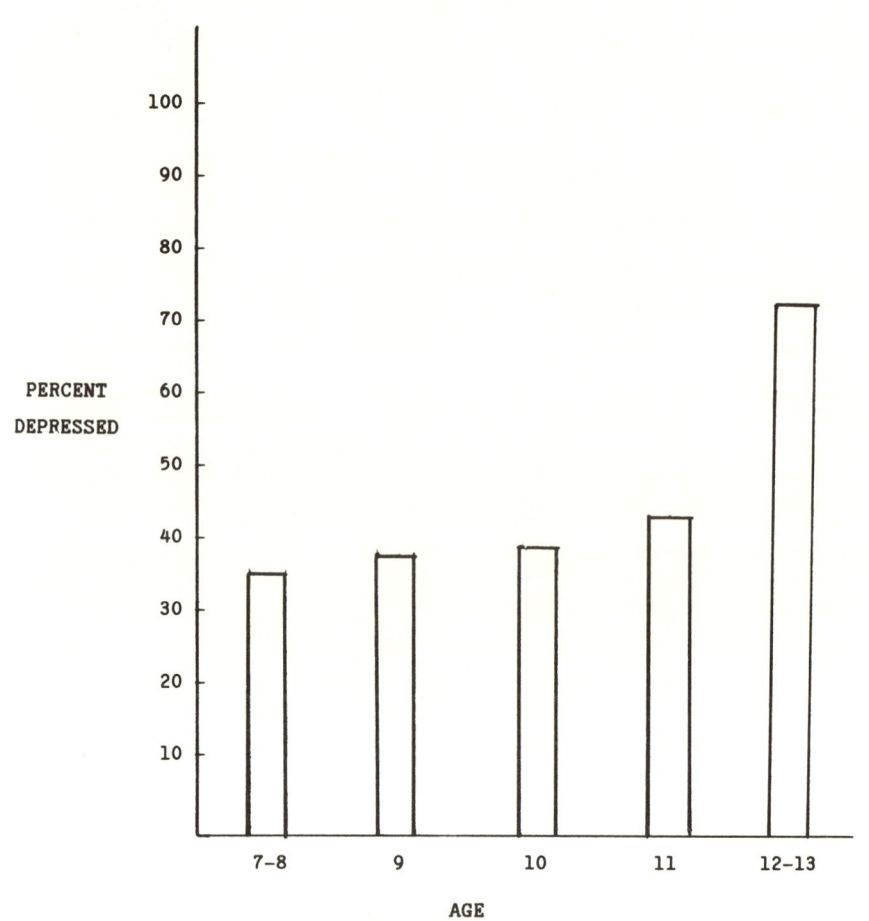

ing to their age into three developmentally meaningful age periods: early school age (seven to eight years, $n = 23$), middle school age (nine to eleven years, $n = 84$), and late school age (twelve to thirteen years, $n = 30$).

Syndrome depression was examined further using the three severity measures of depression. Table 1 compares the mean total scores on the CDI, P-CDI, and CDRS as a function of age. Whereas children in the older age group were rated by parents and clinicians as being significantly more depressed than their younger peers, there was no difference in the self-rated level of depression across ages. Correlations among the three measures were all significant: CDI and P-CDI

Table 1. Comparison of Syndrome Measures as a Function of Age

Measure		7-8	Age 9-11	12-13	F
Children's Depression Inventory					
	M	12.13[a]	9.61[a]	12.50[a]	--
	SD	8.46	7.22	6.64	
Parent—CDI					
	M	9.74[a]	8.89[a]	14.36[a]	5.59*
	SD	8.66	7.32	6.39	
Children's Depression Rating Scale					
	M	38.87[a]	38.86[a]	47.03[b]	6.18*
	SD	10.66	11.81	10.01	

Note: Means having different superscripts differ significantly at *$p < .01$.

($r = .40$, $p < .001$); CDRS and CDI ($r = .69$, $p < .001$); and CDRS and P-CDI ($r = .69$, $p < .001$). These correlations reveal that parents' and children's ratings of depression were moderately and significantly related, although each correlated better with the clinician's judgment of the children's depression.

Comparison of Depressive Symptoms as a Function of Age. The individual symptoms comprising the CDRS were compared as a function of age. Six additional symptoms not specifically defined in the CDRS were also compared. Table 2 reveals the main scores on the individual symptoms for each age group (including depressed and nondepressed children). More than half the symptoms listed are significantly different as a function of age, with the children in the oldest group consistently being rated higher than at least one of the two younger groups.

A careful examination of the symptoms that are rated higher with increasing age reveals that many of these symptoms are associated with the endogenous (biological) subtype of depression. Therefore, we rationally derived a composite endogenous score for each child and contrasted it by age. The endogenous composite item consisted of: pervasive loss of interest, sleep problems, appetite problems, guilt, psychomotor agitation, and hypoactivity. The comparison of this endogenous composite as a function of age revealed a significant difference among the groups [$F(2,134) = 8.36$, $p < .001$], with the oldest group obtaining a significantly higher rating (mean = 10.67), than the two younger groups (means = 8.17 and 8.43, respectively) which did not differ significantly from one another.

Table 2. Comparison of Symptoms as a Function of Age

Children's Depression Rating Scale Symptoms	7-8	Ages 9-11	12-13	F
School problems	3.4[ab]	3.2[a]	3.9[b]	3.87*
Capacity to have fun	2.6[a]	2.7[a]	3.5[b]	6.52**
Social withdrawal	2.3	2.6	2.9	—
Sleep difficulties	2.5	2.6	2.9	—
Appetite problems	1.7[a]	1.9[a]	2.7[b]	9.89***
Fatigue	2.3	2.3	2.9	3.25*
Somatic complaints	2.9	3.0	3.4	—
Irritability	2.6[a]	2.8[a]	3.4[b]	3.44*
Guilt	2.0[a]	1.8[a]	2.5[b]	5.86**
Low self-esteem	3.6[ab]	3.5[a]	4.2[b]	3.11*
Depressed feelings (verbal)	2.6[ab]	2.5[a]	3.1[b]	3.96*
Morbid ideation	1.9	1.5	1.7	—
Suicidal ideation	1.8	1.7	2.1	—
Weeping	2.4	2.1	2.1	—
Depressed affect (nonverbal)	1.7	1.8	2.2	—
Tempo of speech	1.1	1.2	1.3	—
Hypoactivity	1.1[a]	1.5[b]	2.1[c]	9.16***
Additional Symptoms				
Pervasive loss of interest	1.6[a]	1.9[a]	2.5[b]	8.46***
Concentration difficulties	3.4[ab]	3.1[a]	3.7[b]	3.40*
Hopelessness	2.0[a]	2.1[a]	2.7[b]	4.86**
Psychomotor agitation	1.9	1.6	1.5	—
Psychomotor retardation	1.3[a]	1.5[a]	1.9[b]	5.02**
Unresponsive to praise	1.5	1.5	1.5	—

Note: Means not sharing the same superscript differ significantly from one another according to Duncan's multiple-range procedure: *$p < .05$, **$p < .01$, ***$p < .001$.

When only the depressed group is compared, the following symptoms were significantly different by age: morbid ideation [$F(2,61) = 5.72$, $p < .01$], weeping [$F(2,61) = 3.08$, $p < .05$], and hypoactivity ($F(2,61) = 3.07$, $p < .05$). The direction of these differences is particularly interesting. Although hypoactivity was rated as significantly higher in the two older age groups as compared to the youngest group, both morbid ideation and weeping tended to decrease with age, with the youngest group being rated higher than the older two groups for both symptoms. None of the other symptoms were significantly different as a function of age, although for pervasive loss of interest, hopelessness, and appetite problems there was a nonsignificant tendency to increase with age, and for psychomotor agitation a nonsignificant tendency to decrease with age.

Factor Analysis of the Children's Depression Rating Scale. In order to determine that the CDRS was not simply a global measure of general psychopathology or just a compilation of seventeen distinct, unrelated symptoms, a factor analysis was conducted to empirically identify clusters of symptoms that covary. Principle-component factor analysis with orthogonal rotation was used, and only factors with eigenvalues greater than 1.0 were retained. Absolute values of factor loadings are displayed in Table 3, and only loadings of .50 or higher are shown to enhance interpretation of the factors.

The analysis revealed three meaningful factors that may be interpreted as an affective component, an activity component, and a sleep/somatic component. One-way analyses of variance conducted for each factor as a function of age were all significant. Scores for the affective factor [$F(2,134) = 3.50$, $p < .05$], the activity factor [$F(2,134) = 7.14$, $p < .001$], and the sleep/somatic factor [$F(2,134) = 3.07$, $p < .05$] indicate that the older group had significantly higher scores on each factor than one or both of the younger groups.

Discussion

The results of this research indicate that as age increases there is an increase in the frequency of depressive syndrome and also of several of the individual depressive symptoms. These findings are consistent with those found in both clinic (Pearce, 1978) and general population

Table 3. Factor Loading for the Children's Depression Rating Scale (CDRS)

Items	Affective Factor	Activity Factor	Sleep/somatic Factor
School problems		.57	
Capacity to have fun		.53	
Social withdrawal			
Sleep difficulties			.50
Appetite problems		.57	
Fatigue			.61
Somatic complaints			.59
Irritability	.55		
Guilt	.55		
Low self-esteem	.70		
Depressed feelings (verbal)	.70		
Morbid ideation	.50		
Suicidal ideation			
Weeping	.52		
Depressed affect (nonverbal)	.54	.55	
Tempo of speech		.59	
Hypoactivity		.73	
Eigenvalue	7.18	1.53	1.04
Percent of Variance	42.20	9.0	6.1

Note: Only factor loadings over .50 are shown.

studies (Rutter and others, 1976) showing a sharp increase in early adolescence in depressive disorder as well as in the individual symptoms of misery, depression, and self-depreciation. Although this increase has been found for both sexes, it is apparently much more marked in girls (Rutter, in press).

In the present study, the symptoms that tended to increase as a function of age were: appetite problems, hypoactivity, pervasive loss of interest, capacity to have fun, guilt, hopelessness, irritability, fatigue, problems at school, difficulty concentrating, depressed feelings, and low self-esteem. Symptoms that tended to decrease significantly with age (among the depressed children only) were morbid ideation and weeping. There was a nonsignificant tendency, however, for these symptoms as well as psychomotor agitation to decrease with age for the whole sample.

It is interesting to speculate within a developmental framework as to the possible reasons for the developmental changes observed. Rutter (in press) outlined several potential explanations for the increase in depressive symptomatology with adolescence, including hormonal changes associated with puberty, genetic factors, frequency of environmental stressors, degree of either vulnerability or protective factors, the cognitive set associated with learned helplessness, and developmental changes in children's concepts and expression of affect. Irritability, for example, has been found to be associated with depression during the premenstrual phase of a woman's cycle (Sommer, 1978), and this is more likely to be seen in girls who have reached or are approaching puberty.

There also was an increase with age in verbalized depressed feelings, although not in observed nonverbal depressed affect. Early writers about childhood depression (for example, Cytryn and McKnew, 1972; Glaser, 1967; Malmquist, 1971) manufactured the concept of *masked depression* to explain the observation that young children typically do not verbalize depressive feelings, although Malmquist (1971) recognized that even though children do not complain of sadness, they often present a behavioral and nonverbal expressive picture that conveys it. More recently, developmental psychopathologists (Cicchetti and Schneider-Rosen, in press; Rutter, in press) have suggested that there are developmental changes in children's concepts of emotions and in their ability to express affect that may account for the increased verbalization of depressed affect with age observed in the present study.

Another classic symptom of depression that correlated with age was low self-esteem. The ability to judge oneself is dependent on the individual having a self-representation, the capacity to evaluate oneself according to one's own standards, and the ability to consider the perspective of others (Kovacs, in press). The developmental literature supports the notion that self-understanding (Damon and Hart, 1982), self-evaluation (Mullener and Laird, 1971), and social perspective-taking (Selman and others, 1977) undergo progressive refinement and differentiation with age. With developing cognitive capacity, children can think abstractly, rather than concretely. Thus, they can use psychological dimensions rather than physical characteristics and behaviors to describe themselves (Damon and Hart, 1982; Lively and Bromley, 1973). In addition, they develop the affective capacity to evaluate themselves in terms of positive and negative (Wylie, 1979) which may account for the increasing low self-esteem observed among the older children.

Consistent with the findings of earlier studies of childhood depression (for example, McConville and others, 1973; Ushakov and Girich, 1972), the present study also found an increase with age in the symptom of guilt. Because children have less potent notions of personal responsibility and only gradually acquire standards of right and wrong, it is not surprising that the expression of guilt changes with age. In an attributional analysis of emotional development, Weiner and Graham (in press) reported a developmental trend in the nature of guilt expressed in children. Younger children expressed guilt with respect to uncontrollable or accidental outcomes. Older children endorsed guilt for controllable outcomes involving intentionality. This latter type of guilt, resembling "personal responsibility," distinguishes the childhood symptom of guilt from the "universal responsibility" characteristic of adult depression (Abramson and others, 1978).

The final symptom of interest from a developmental perspective is hopelessness. The experience of hopelessness is largely dependent on the cognitive capacity to formulate expectations and to comprehend the temporal perspective of future. Both capacities are limited among younger children (Bemporad and Wilson, 1978; Cicchetti and Schneider-Rosen, in press; Rie, 1966). In general, school-age children have shorter future orientations than adolescents and adults (Doob, 1971). Moreover, younger children's self-descriptions tend to be present-oriented, and it is not until adolescence that individuals express personal continuity in the sense of a past and future self (Damon and Hart, 1982). Therefore, the experience of hopelessness will presumably parallel the development of a more comprehensive temporal orientation that includes a sense of future.

One symptom that is noteworthy because of the apparent lack of increase with age in the present sample was suicidal ideation. Statistics show that actual suicides are quite rare in early childhood (Shaffer,

1974). The number increases significantly during adolescence. There is little data, however, on the developmental progression of suicidal ideation per se. Although there was a nonsignificant tendency in this study for the older children's scores to be higher, suicidal ideation tended to be a relatively rare symptom across the entire sample. This may be due, in part, to the fact that all of the children in this sample were under age fourteen, the age at which suicide tends to increase significantly (Shaffer and Fisher, 1981). An interesting anecdotal point is that the two children in the present sample who had made suicide attempts were both in the oldest age group (ages 13.1 and 12.8).

It may also initially seem unexpected that morbid ideation tended to decrease with age. Poznanski and others (1979) separated suicidal and morbid ideation on the CDRS because morbid ideation occurs both with and without suicidal ideation. The present results seem to confirm that these factors do indeed measure somewhat different constructs that tend to differ developmentally. Renshaw (1973) suggested that preoccupation with morbidity among young children reflects their rich fantasy life and very crude conceptualization of death. Moreover, the wording of the morbid ideation item on the CDRS may be encouraging the younger child's greater tendency to worry, particularly about significant others getting hurt or dying (Ushakov and Girich, 1972).

Other symptoms that did not differ significantly as a function of age (although the means were all in the direction of increasing with age) were social withdrawal, somatic complaints, and sleep difficulties. It is interesting that the former two symptoms are not part of the typical adult criteria for defining depression, but do tend to be associated with depression in children. Children often present somatic complaints instead of more overt expressions of unhappiness. It is easier for children to recognize and express physical complaints than it is for them to express the negative affect of sadness. Despite the fact that these symptoms did not differ significantly as a function of age when examined individually, they did each comprise an important part of the three syndromal factors — affect, activity, and sleep/somatic disorder — which all did differ significantly with age.

Not only were there developmental differences in the overall syndrome as well as the specific symptoms of depression, but there also were age differences in both the rationally defined cluster of endogenous symptoms and the empirically derived factors. An important critique of Lefkowitz and Burton's (1978) conclusion that depressive symptoms are so prevalent that they cannot be considered pathological was that they neglected to consider the prevalence of the syndrome or constellation of symptoms (Costello, 1980). The present study examined individual symptoms, subclusters of symptoms, and the entire syndrome, although not the nosologic disorder, from a developmental perspective. Results indicate that depression in children as measured by the CDRS is neither simply a global psychopathological entity nor a compilation of seventeen independent symptoms. Rather, childhood depression appears to consist of three meaningful factors including affective, activity, and sleep/somatic components, all of which tend to increase as a function of age. The results of the factor analysis should be considered with caution, however, until they can be cross-validated in a new sample.

Despite the trend toward an increase in frequency and severity of depressive symptoms and syndrome with increasing age, it is noteworthy nonetheless that a proportion of the seven- and eight-year-old children manifested the depressive syndrome. This is consistent with earlier studies (McConville and others, 1973; Ushakov and Girich, 1972) that found the beginnings of a depression-like syndrome in children over the age of seven. In order to observe more clearcut developmental differences it would be useful to expand the age ranges at both ends to include a sample of preschool children and adolescents.

Advantages of the CDRS. An important reason why an adultlike syndrome could be seen in even the youngest children is that the methods of assessment described here were chosen intentionally to discover the child manifestations of the so-called adult symptoms. The CDRS as used in the present investigation was designed with a developmental perspective in mind; how the questions are asked and how the items are defined take into consideration the limitations of the developing linguistic, cognitive, and semantic capacities of children. For example, the CDRS includes both a verbal and nonverbal item of depressed affect, allowing for the young child's tendency away from overt expression of depressive affect. Moreover, the questions regarding self-esteem, capacity to have fun, guilt, and hypoactivity all were phrased using age-appropriate language. The criteria used to define these symptoms were broad enough to incorporate possible developmental differences in their manifestation. For example, the self-esteem item asks about specific areas of the self such as appearance, intelligence, and relationship with peers, rather than a general question about whether or not the child likes him or herself which elicits the response, "Yes, of course." By asking the child to respond to concrete questions about particular areas, the clinician can then make a judgment regarding the overall evaluative tone of the descriptors.

The developmental orientation of the CDRS is also evident in its inclusion of social withdrawal and physical complaints—symptoms not typically part of the adult disorder. Moreover, the item assessing concentration difficulties has been broadened to include a general change in school performance that may or may not be associated with concentration problems. The new and altered symptoms allow for the possibility that the childhood form of the disorder may differ from the adult syndrome both in terms of the symptoms included as well as the precise criteria used to define them. By broadening the operational criteria defining the symptoms as well as the specific language used to assess them, it may be possible to observe developmentally appropriate manifestations of the syndrome.

CDRS ratings are made by a clinician who uses all available information—including the children, parents, teachers, and records. It is possible that, if we were to examine the developmental progression of depressive symptoms with age as a function of the informant, very different results might emerge. The developmental limitations regarding children's cognitive and linguistic capacities might become even more apparent if we were to conduct the analyses presented in this study for the child-reported data only. It is interesting, however, in the present study, that one child self-report measure used (CDI) showed no significant differences as a function of age, whereas the parent version of the same measure (P-CDI) did differ significantly with age. It is possible that parents' reporting of symptoms are influenced by their own beliefs and expectations about their children's capacities. The issue of the discrepancy between parent and child report has been discussed elsewhere (see Garber, 1983; Weissman and others, 1980), and has important implications for the assessment and classification of psychopathology in children.

Finally, a few caveats concerning the generalizability and interpretability of the results presented here should be mentioned. First, these data were collected on a sample of girls only, and therefore obviously do not reflect the developmental progression of depression in boys. A similar type of study needs to be conducted on a male sample. Second, these data reflect cross-sectional age differences in different children rather than longitudinal differences among the same children, and thus do not represent the developmental course of depressive symptomatology. Finally, the clinician's ratings of the CDRS were made by only one judge and therefore need to be checked for reliability with a second independent rater. This analysis is currently being conducted.

Summary

The results of this study are consistent with the developmental perspective that shows significant changes with age—influenced by developmental changes in cognitive, linguistic, and socioemotional capacities—in children's expression of depressive symptomatology. Moreover, by broadening the diagnostic criteria and using assessment procedures that are consistent with children's age-appropriate capacities, we will be better able to detect the manner in which the expression of symptoms alters with development. A thorough knowledge of normal developmental processes will enable us to construct the age-appropriate classifications and to develop the age-appropriate assessment methodologies necessary for an adequate understanding of the impact that children's developing capacities may have on the etiology and phenomenology of depressive symptoms over the course of development.

References

Abramson, L. Y., Seligman, M. E. P., and Teasdale, J. D. "Learned Helplessness in Humans: Critique and Reformulation." *Journal of Abnormal Psychology,* 1978, *87,* 49-74.

Achenbach, T. M. "The Classification of Children's Psychiatric Symptoms: A Factor-Analytic Study." *Psychological Monograph,* 1966, *80* (7, Whole No. 615).

Achenbach, T. M. "The Child Behavior Profile: I. Boys Aged 6-11." *Journal of Consulting and Clinical Psychology,* 1978, *47,* 223-233.

Achenbach, T. M. "The Child Behavior Profile: II. Boys Aged 12-16 and Girls Aged 6-11 and 12-16." *Journal of Consulting and Clinical Psychology,* 1979, *47,* 223-233.

Ainsworth, M., Blehar, M., Waters, E., and Wall, S. *Patterns of Attachment.* Hillsdale, N.J.: Erlbaum, 1978.

American Psychiatric Association. *Diagnostic and Statistical Manual of Mental Disorders.* (3rd ed.) Washington, D.C.: American Psychiatric Association, 1980.

Anthony, E. J. "Depression and Children." In E. Borrows (Ed.), *Handbook of Studies on Depression.* Princeton, N.J.: Excerpta Medica, 1977.

Beck, A. T. *Depression: Causes and Treatment.* New York: Harper & Row, 1967.

Bemporad, J. R., and Wilson, A. "A Developmental Approach to Depression in Childhood and Adolescence." *Journal of the American Academy of Psychoanalysis,* 1978, *6,* 325-352.

Brumback, R. A., Dietz-Schmidt, G., and Weinberg, W. A. "Depression in Children Referred to an Educational Diagnostic Center: Diagnosis and Treatment and Analysis of Criteria and Literature Review." *Diseases of the Nervous System,* 1977, *7,* 529-535.

Brumback, R. A., and Weinberg, W. A. "Mania in Childhood. II Therapeutic Trial of Lithium Carbonate and Further Description of Manic Depressive Illness in Children." *American Journal of Disorders of the Child,* 1979, *131,* 1122-1126.

Carlson, G. A., and Strober, M. "Affective Disorder in Adolescence." *Psychiatric Clinics of North America,* 1979, *2,* 511-533.

Cicchetti, D., and Pogge-Hesse, P. "Possible Contributions of the Study of Organically

Retarded Persons to Developmental Theory." In E. Zigler and D. Balla (Eds.), *The Developmental-Difference Controversy.* Hillsdale, N.J.: Erlbaum, 1982.

Cicchetti, D., and Schneider-Rosen, K. "An Organizational Approach to Childhood Depression." In M. Rutter, C. Izard, and P. B. Read (Eds.), *Depression in Childhood: Developmental Perspectives.* New York: Guilford Press, in press.

Commins, S., and Heisler, A. B. "Depression in Children and Adolescents." *Pediatric Annals,* 1980, *9,* 263-268.

Costello, C. G. "Childhood Depression: Three Basic but Questionable Assumptions in the Lefkowitz and Burton Critique." *Psychological Bulletin,* 1980, *87,* 185-190.

Cytryn, L., and McKnew, D. H. "Proposed Classification of Childhood Depression." *American Journal of Psychiatry,* 1972, *129,* 149-155.

Cytryn, L., McKnew, D. H., and Bunney, W. E. "Diagnosis of Depression in Children: A Reassessment." *American Journal of Psychiatry,* 1980, *137,* 22-25.

Damon, W., and Hart, D. "The Development of Self-Understanding from Infancy Through Adolescence." *Child Development,* 1982, *53,* 841-864.

"Depressive and Manic Sickness in Childhood." *The Nervous Child,* 1952, *9,* 309-422.

Doob, L. W. *Patterning of Time.* New Haven: Yale University Press, 1971.

Engel, G., and Reichsman, F. "Spontaneous and Experimentally Induced Depressions in an Infant with a Gastric Fistula." *Journal of American Psychoanalytic Association,* 1956, *9,* 428-456.

Flavell, J. H. *Cognitive Development.* Englewood Cliffs, N.J.: Prentice-Hall, 1977.

Garber, J. "Parents' Ratings of Their Children's Depression." Paper presented at the Annual Convention of the American Psychological Association, August 1983, Anaheim, California.

Garber, J. "Classification of Childhood Psychopathology: A Developmental Perspective." *Child Development,* 1984, *55,* 30-48.

Gittelman-Klein, R. "Definitional and Methodological Issues Concerning Depressive Illness in Children." In J. G. Schulterbrandt and A. Raskin (Eds.), *Depression in Childhood.* New York: Raven Press, 1977.

Glaser, K. "Masked Depression in Children and Adolescents." *Annual Progress in Child Psychiatry and Child Development,* 1967, *1,* 345-355.

Greenspan, S. I., Lourie, R. S., and Nover, R. A. "A Developmental Approach to the Classification of Psychopathology in Infancy and Early Childhood." In J. Noshpitz (Ed.), *Handbook of Child Psychiatry.* New York: Basic Books, 1979.

Hamilton, M. "A Rating Scale for Depression." *Journal of Neurology, Neurosurgery, and Psychiatry,* 1969, *23,* 56-61.

Herjanic, B., Herjanic, M., Brown, F., and Wheatt, T. "Are Children Reliable Reporters?" *Journal of Abnormal Child Psychology,* 1975, *3,* 41-48.

Kanner, L. *Child Psychiatry.* (3rd ed.) Springfield, Ill.: Thomas, 1957.

Kovacs, M. "Rating Scales to Assess Depression in School-Aged Children." *Acta Paedopsychiatrica,* 1981, *46,* 305-315.

Kovacs, M. "A Developmental Perspective on Methods and Measures in the Assessment of Depressive Disorders: The Clinical Interview." In M. Rutter, C. E. Izard, and P. B. Read (Eds.), *Depression in Childhood: Developmental Perspectives.* New York: Guilford Press, in press.

Kovacs, M., and Beck, A. T. "An Empirical-Clinical Approach Toward a Definition of Childhood Depression." In J. G. Schulterbrandt and A. Raskin (Eds.), *Depression in Childhood: Diagnosis, Treatment, and Conceptual Models.* New York: Raven Press, 1977.

Lefkowitz, M. M., and Burton, N. "Childhood Depression: A Critique of the Concept." *Psychological Bulletin,* 1978, *85,* 716-726.

Livesly, W. J., and Bromley, D. B. *Person Perception in Childhood and Adolescence.* New York: Wiley, 1973.
McConville, B. J., Boag, L. C., and Purohit, A. P. "Three Types of Childhood Depression." *Canadian Psychiatric Association Journal,* 1973, *18,* 133-138.
Mahler, M. S. "On Sadness and Grief in Infancy and Childhood." *Psychoanalytic Study of the Child,* 1961, *16,* 332-354.
Malmquist, C. P. "Depressions in Childhood and Adolescence." *New England Journal of Medicine,* 1971, *284,* 887-893.
Matas, L., Arend, R. A., and Sroufe, L. A. "Continuity of Adaptation in the Second Year: The Relationship Between Quality of Attachment and Later Competence." *Child Development,* 1978, *49,* 547-556.
Mullener, N., and Laird, J. D. "Some Developmental Changes in the Organization of Self-Evaluations." *Developmental Psychology,* 1971, *5,* 233-236.
Pearce, J. B. "The Recognition of Depressive Disorder in Children." *Journal of the Royal Society of Medicine,* 1978, *71,* 494-500.
Piaget, J. *The Construction of Reality in the Child.* New York: Basic Books, 1954.
Poznanski, E. O., Cook, S. C., and Carroll, B. J. "A Depression Rating Scale for Children." *Pediatrics,* 1979, *64,* 442-450.
Poznanski, E. O., and Zrull, J. P. "Childhood Depression: Clinical Characteristics of Overtly Depressed Children." *Archives of General Psychiatry,* 1970, *23,* 8-15.
Puig-Antich, J., and Chambers, W. *The Schedule of Affective Disorders and Schizophrenia for Children (K-SADS).* Unpublished manuscript, 1979.
Puig-Antich, J., Blau, S., Marx, N., Greenhill, L. L., and Chambers, W. "Pre-Pubertal Major Depressive Disorder: A Pilot Study." *Journal of the American Academy of Child Psychiatry,* 1978, *17,* 695-707.
Renshaw, D. C. "Depression in the Young." *Journal of the American Medical Woman's Association,* 1973, *28,* 542-546.
Rie, H. E. "Depression in Childhood: A Survey of Some Pertinent Contributions." *Journal of the American Academy of Child Psychiatry,* 1966, *5,* 653-685.
Robins, E., and Guze, S. B. "Classification of Affective Disorders: The Primary-Secondary, the Endogenous-Reactive, and the Neurotic-Psychotic Concepts." In T. A. Williams, M. M. Katz, and J. A. Shields (Eds.), *Recent Advances in the Psychobiology of the Depressive Illnesses.* Chevy Chase, Md.: U.S. Department of Health, Education, and Welfare, 1969.
Rochlin, G. "The Loss Complex." *Journal of the American Psychoanalytic Association,* 1959, *7,* 299-316.
Rutter, M. "Emotional Development." In M. Rutter (Ed.), *Scientific Foundations of Developmental Psychiatry.* London: Heinemann, 1980.
Rutter, M. "The Developmental Psychopathology of Depression: Issues and Perspectives." In M. Rutter, C. E. Izard, and P. B. Read (Eds.), *Depression in Childhood: Developmental Perspectives.* New York: Guilford Press, in press.
Rutter, M., Graham, P., Chadwick, D., and Yale, W. "Adolescent Turmoil: Factor or Fiction?" *Journal of Child Psychology and Psychiatry,* 1976, *17,* 35-36.
Rutter, M., Tizard, J., and Whitmore, K. (Eds.). *Education, Health, and Behavior.* London: Longman, 1970.
Sandler, J., and Joffe, W. G. "Notes on Childhood Depression." *International Journal of Psychoanalysis,* 1965, *46,* 88-96.
Santostefano, S. "Beyond Nosology: Prognosis from the Viewpoint of Development." In H. E. Rie (Ed.), *Perspectives in Child Psychopathology.* Chicago: Aldine, 1971.
Saussure, R. de. "J. B. Felix Descuret." *The Psychoanalytic Study of the Child,* 1947, *2,* 417-426.

Selman, R. L., Jaquette, D., and Redman, L. D. "Interpersonal Awareness in Children Toward an Integration of Developmental and Clinical Child Psychology." *American Journal of Orthopsychiatry,* 1977, *47,* 264-274.

Shaffer, D., "Suicide in Childhood and Early Adolescence." *Journal of Child Psychology and Psychiatry,* 1974, *15,* 275-292.

Shaffer, D., and Fisher, P. "The Epidemiology of Suicide in Children and Young Adolescents." *Journal of the American Academy of Child Psychiatry,* 1981, *20,* 545-565.

Sommer, B. B. "Stress and Menstrual Distress." *Journal of Human Stress,* 1978, *4,* 5-10, 41-47.

Spitz, R. "Anaclitic Depression." *Psychoanalytic Study of the Child,* 1946, *2,* 113-117.

Sroufe, L. A. "The Coherence of Individual Development: Early Care, Attachment, and Subsequent Development Issues." *American Psychologist,* 1979, *34,* 834-841.

Sroufe, L. A., and Rutter, M. "The Domain of Development Psychopathology." *Child Development,* 1984, *55,* 17-29.

Toolan, J. M. "Depression in Children and Adolescents." *American Journal of Orthopsychiatry,* 1962, *32,* 404-414.

Ushakov, G. K., and Girich, Y. P. "Special Features of Psychogenic Depressions in Children and Adolescents." In A. Annell (Ed.), *Depressive States in Childhood and Adolescence.* Stockholm: Almquist & Wiksell, 1972.

Weinberg, W. A., Rutman, J., Sullivan, L., Penick, E. C., and Dietz, S. G. "Depression in Children Referred to an Educational Diagnostic Center: Diagnosis and Treatment." *Journal of Pediatrics,* 1973, *83,* 1065-1072.

Weiner, B., and Graham, S. "An Attributional Approach to Emotional Development." In C. E. Izard, J. Kogan, and R. Zajonc (Eds.), *Emotions, Cognition, and Behavior.* New York: Cambridge University Press, in press.

Weissman, M. M., and Myers, J. K. "Affective Disorder in the U.S. Urban Community." *Archives of General Psychiatry,* 1978, *35,* 1304-1311.

Weissman, M. M., Orvaschel, H., and Padian, N. "Children's Symptom and Social Functioning Self-Report Scales: Comparison of Mother's and Children's Reports." *Journal of Nervous and Mental Diseases,* 1980, *168,* 736-740.

Werner, H. *Comparative Psychology of Mental Development.* New York: International Universities Press, 1948.

Wylie, R. C. *The Self Concept: Theory and Research on Selected Topics.* Vol. 2. (rev. ed.) Lincoln: University of Nebraska Press, 1979.

Judy Garber is a graduate student in clinical child psychology at the University of Minnesota.

Traditional hypotheses regarding developmental parameters and characteristics of the depressive disorders in children are difficult to verify empirically; in fact, the study of developmental psychopathology may require novel conceptual strategies.

Developmental Stage and the Expression of Depressive Disorders in Children: An Empirical Analysis

Maria Kovacs
Stana L. Paulauskas

The existence and significance of the depressive disorders in childhood is supported by a growing body of empirical research. Several studies have demonstrated, for example, that school-aged depressed youngsters can be identified and diagnosed according to the Research Diagnostic Criteria (Spitzer and others, 1978) and the recent Diagnostic and Statistical Manual of Mental Disorders (DSM-III, American Psychiatric Association, 1980; Carlson and Cantwell, 1980, 1982a; Kovacs and

This research project has been supported by Grant Number MH-33990 from the National Institute of Mental Health, Health and Human Services Administration; partial support has been provided by Clinical Center Grant Number MH-30915.

Joseph Verducci of the Department of Statistics at Ohio State University has provided statistical consultation.

others, 1984a, 1984b; Puig-Antich and others, 1978, 1982). It has been also established that depressed children suffer from their disorders far longer than hitherto thought (Kovacs and others, 1984a); are likely to have educational as well as social difficulties (Kovacs and others, 1984a; Puig-Antich and Weston, 1983); and can be treated effectively with antidepressant medication (Preskorn and others, 1982; Puig-Antich and others, 1979).

Most recent investigations, however, have bypassed issues of developmental psychology and have relied on diagnostic and assessment methods that were originally designed for adults. Therefore, it is unlikely that the findings will be accepted readily or unequivocally. For example, Herzog and Rathbun (1982) and Malmquist (1983) have already criticized the current diagnostic system because it does not take into account that the child's stage of development influences the expression of the depressive syndrome. Traditional arguments for a relationship between developmental stage and depression in the child (Conners, 1976; Kovacs and Beck, 1977; Lefkowitz and Burton, 1978) may provide the basis for more specific reservations about the existing research. Because developmental concerns have long dominated the field of childhood depression, an overview of the various vantage points is highly pertinent to the present chapter.

The historically earliest developmental stance on childhood depression derives from classic psychoanalytic theory. According to this paradigm, melancholia cannot exist without introjected hostility or pathological guilt (Gaylin, 1968). However, guilt is allegedly absent from the child's affective repertoire by virtue of the fact that his or her psychosexual development is incomplete. Thus, as Rochlin (1959) stated, "classical depression, a superego phenomenon, as we psychoanalytically understand the disorder, does not occur in childhood" (p. 299).

From the perspective of ego-analytic theory, however (Bibring, 1953; Jacobson, 1953), object loss and negative self-esteem are central to depression. It is assumed that the characteristics of these two factors vary across the age span. In contrast to the adult, the child presumably perceives and reacts to loss as a temporary phenomenon and cannot sustain a negative self-view. Therefore, from an ego-analytic stance, depression in the juvenile years is plausible, but it is ostensibly less persistent and severe than it is in adults (Bemporad, 1978; Makita, 1973; Rie, 1966).

The final developmental position on the issue of childhood depression has been an eclectic one. Its representatives have utilized combinations of psychological and biological constructs to argue that developmental stage determines the manifest symptom picture. For example, insofar as the juvenile's perceptions are present oriented and context bound, he or she is presumably unlikely to experience hopelessness or self-denigration (McConville and others, 1973; Rie, 1966; Siomopoulos and Inamdar, 1979). Instead, feelings of loneliness and isolation may predominate (McConville and others, 1973). Others have proposed that, because the child is innately hedonistic and cannot tolerate despair, he or she will defend the self against the subjective experience of depression by "acting out" (Cytryn and McKnew, 1972; Glaser, 1968). Herzog and Rathbun's (1982) diagnostic schema and Makita's (1973) observations imply that somatosexual maturity also affect the manifestation of the depressive syndrome. Accordingly, the classic depressive symptoms should be most evident subsequent to the onset of puberty.

The mechanisms whereby pubertal stage may mediate the phenomenology of depression in children have not been specified. However, as already exemplified above, from current psychological theories one can generate hypotheses about how developmental stage influences clinical presentation. For instance, Piaget's theory (1950) suggests that notions of hopelessness and worthlessness entail formal operational thinking. Therefore, it can be hypothesized that these two symptoms should not be evident among depressed youngsters who are at the preoperational or concrete operational stages of cognitive development.

Hypotheses about the age at which certain depressive symptoms emerge can be also derived from the empirical literature on the unfolding of other presumably pertinent capacities. For example, there is considerable documentation showing that normal children go through developmental changes in their understanding and characterization of the emotions (Schwartz and Trabasso, in press), their temporal perspective (Wessman and Gorman, 1977), self-conception (Damon and Hart, 1982) and interpersonal, social-cognitive system (Shantz, 1975).

Nonetheless, in spite of continued speculations along developmental lines about the expression and classification of childhood depression (Herzog and Rathbun, 1982; Malmquist, 1983), few of the propositions have been tested empirically (Glasberg and Aboud, 1981; Paulauskas, 1983). And even the correlation between chronological age and the changing phenomenology of the syndrome has been barely explored (Carlson and Cantwell, 1982b).

In this chapter, therefore, we describe an empirical examination of the developmental-stage mediation of depression in clinically referred school-aged children. Two parameters of development were studied: cognitive development and somatosexual (pubertal) development. To remedy shortcomings in the existing literature, the subjects were diagnosed according to operational criteria; moreover, standardized measures were used to quantify the pertinent independent variables.

The selection of an appropriate test of cognitive development presented a problem for a number of reasons. First, it has been documented that performance can vary across tasks that are theoretically alike but are dissimilar in content (Rubin, 1973, 1978). On the other hand, it has been also suggested that the use of only one task may not provide a true measure of the child's capacity (Gelman, 1978). Furthermore, in view of the diverse cognitive, social, and personal complaints or symptoms that constitute much of the phenomenology of depression (Beck, 1967), we were uncertain which cognitive domain was heuristically most relevant to the study of this disorder. Therefore, we assessed three facets of cognition: interpersonal reasoning, impersonal reasoning, and understanding of self-identity. The results were then combined into an overall index of the child's stage of cognitive development.

The goal of the investigation was to examine whether characteristics of the depressive disorder and the type of manifest symptoms conform to developmental expectations. By definition (American Psychiatric Association, 1980), a *depressive disorder* is a *syndrome* (a cluster of characteristic symptoms and signs) that meets psychiatric diagnostic criteria. A *symptom* refers to one specific complaint or manifestation of the disorder.

It was assumed that stage of cognitive development has its greatest explanatory power with respect to the presence or absence of psychosocial symptoms of depression (hopelessness, self-deprecation, inability to experience pleasure, among others). On the other hand, stage of puberty, as an index of biological maturation, was presumed to be most pertinent to the mediation of vegetative or psychomotor symptoms (for example, disturbances in sleep, appetite, and energy level). Both developmental variables were expected to influence the duration and the chronicity of the depressive disorder.

Method

The data were gathered as part of a larger, ongoing, longitudinal nosologic study of two age-matched cohorts: a group of depressed children and a nondepressed psychiatric comparison group. The overall design and the specific methods have been described (Kovacs and others, 1984a).

Subjects were recruited sequentially (as they became available) and were assessed four times during the first year of their study participation and twice a year subsequently. At each assessment, a multifaceted battery of tests was administered to the child and the parent.

Symptomatic and diagnostic data were gathered in direct interviews by experienced and specially trained clinical psychologists and psychiatric social workers independent of and blind to the results of cognitive- and pubertal-stage assessment. The cognitive tasks were administered and scored by trained research assistants who held bachelor's or master's degrees. Pubertal stage was determined by a pediatrician during a brief physical examination. The clinical and diagnostic assessments were repeated at each research contact, whereas cognitive and pubertal stages were determined once a year.

Subjects. The present chapter concerns only the depressed children from our study, not the comparison group. The children were referrals to the University of Pittsburgh School of Medicine's child psychiatric and general pediatric outpatient clinics who met the following initial criteria: eight to thirteen years old, no evidence of mental retardation or major systemic medical illness, ambulatory psychiatric and medical status, and living with at least one parent or legal guardian. At the intake research evaluation, or within the following six months, these children also met DSM-III psychiatric diagnostic criteria for major depressive disorder, dysthymic disorder, or adjustment disorder with depressed mood (American Psychiatric Association, 1980).

We report on the first eighty cases in the depressed sample. At study entry, thirty-two children had the diagnosis of major depressive disorder, twenty-one had dysthymic disorder, eleven met diagnostic criteria for both major depressive and dysthymic disorders, and sixteen cases had adjustment disorder with depressed mood. There were thirty-eight girls (48 percent) and forty-two boys (53 percent); 45 percent of the sample was in the ten- to eleven-year-old age range; mean age was 11.27 years. The sample was racially mixed with a preponderance of Caucasian children (58 percent). Based on Hollingshead's (1957) index of socioeconomic status (SES), 63 percent of the group was of middle SES (II, III, and IV), but there was an overrepresentation of the lowest SES level (V—31 percent). Only 29 percent of the sample was living with both biological parents; therefore the overwhelming majority of the children were from broken homes.

At study intake, 66 percent of the youngsters were attending only regular classes at their schools; 30 percent were receiving part- or full-time remedial instruction; 4 percent were in accelerated learning programs. According to their WISC-R vocabulary subtest test age, 78 percent scored within the range that corresponded to the study's chronological age cutoff (eight to thirteen years); 9 percent tested lower than eight years of age, and 14 percent had a test age that exceeded fourteen years. A notable portion of the sample had failed one or more grades (30 percent) and 27 percent had a history of one or more school suspensions. Finally, 32 percent had previous outpatient treatment for emotional and behavioral problems.

Clinical Evaluation and Diagnosis. As described in detail elsewhere (Kovacs and others, 1984a), psychiatric diagnoses were determined by consensus among members of our team of research clinicians. The diagnoses were based on the symptomatic results of the semi-structured Interview Schedule for Children (ISC, Kovacs, 1983), anamnestic data, qualitative clinical history, and the results of standardized psychometric tests, when needed. The diagnoses conformed to the rules of the DSM-III. The same procedure was followed at every research visit.

The semi-structured psychiatric interview (ISC) is a standardized symptom-oriented schedule. It includes the most common symptoms and signs of the depressive syndrome and facilitates their quantification. At each assessment, the ISC was administered by one of our research clinicians.

Using the ISC, a clinician first interviewed the parent about the child—the resultant data constituted the "parent-interview" symptom ratings. Then, the same clinician interviewed the child alone about him- or herself with the same ISC, producing the "child-interview" symptom ratings. Additionally, the clinician gave a third rating for each item based on a synthesis of information from the parent and the child. On the ISC, the symptom ratings were entered sequentially as the interview progressed and by means of predefined severity scales. Diagnostic decisions were based on the clinician's synthesized symptom ratings, whereas determination of the onset and duration of a disorder was based primarily on data obtained from the parents.

Pubertal Stage Determination. The child's pubertal stage was assessed by pediatric examination according to the guidelines of Tanner (1962). The Tanner score can range from I—prepubertal genitalia—to V—adult genitalia. The information can be analyzed as a "continuous" variable or can be dichotomized into prepubertal stage (Tanner I) versus various stages of puberty up to full somatosexual maturity (Tanner II through V).

Cognitive Stage Determination. Three tasks were administered in a randomized order, the results of which were then combined into a global index. The Combinations Task and the Personal Identity Interview were preceded by a practice period to teach the child the pertinent rules. To facilitate scoring, the Combinations and the Interpersonal

Reasoning Tasks were tape-recorded and transcribed. The protocol for each task was scored independently by two scorers; disagreements were resolved by consensus.

The Combinations Task (CT). The ability to consider all possible combinations of relevant variables in a given problem situation—one of the components of formal operational thinking (Piaget and Inhelder, 1975)—was assessed using sets of six differently colored toy cars; instructions were adapted from Goodnow (1962). Based on the child's actual productions with the stimulus set and his or her oral account of how the problem was solved, the subject's performance can be categorized into one of three stages: preoperational (I), concrete operational (II), or formal operational (III).

The Interpersonal Reasoning Task (IRT). The IRT exemplifies a social dilemma that derives from Selman's (1980) model of interpersonal inference. We selected a "Person Interview" task—the Ping-Pong story—that taps the construct of subjectivity (Selman and others, 1979). The interviewer tells the story and then poses questions to elicit the child's conception of the interrelationship of one's feelings, thoughts, and motives in relation to an interpersonal situation. According to the scoring manual (Selman and others, 1979), the subject's oral productions can be categorized at one of five stages that range from zero (the inability to recognize that a person can be happy and sad at the same time, for example) to four (for instance, the ability to integrate and reconcile different and potentially conflicting feelings and motives).

The Personal Identity Interview (PII). Mohr (1978) developed the PII based on the thesis that self-understanding develops in a sequence of stages similar to the unfolding of other cognitive capacities. During the PII, questions are posed about the continuity or discontinuity of the self—for example, "What will or will not change about you when you grow up?" The child's oral responses can be classified at one of three levels: externally or physically oriented conceptualizations (I), behavioral or activity-based conceptualizations (II), and "internal" or abstract, trait-type attributions (III).

To determine the global index of cognitive-developmental stage, scores on each of the tasks were dichotomized. On Selman's IRT, scores of zero, one, and two were collapsed into one category that was labeled "not integrative," and its opposite—scores of three and four—was labeled "integrative." On the Piagetian CT, scores were collapsed into the category of "not formal" (stages I and II) versus "formal" (stage III). On Mohr's PII, the dichotomy was between "not internal" (Stages I and II) and "internal" (stage III). We assumed a similarity between the ability to integrate and synthesize different feelings and motives, the stage of formal operations, and internal attributions of personal identity. Performance at the lower levels was also assumed to be structurally similar. Using the Selman IRT as the primary marker or classifier, we arrived at the following cognitive-stage designations that were used in this study:

- *Primarily concrete* (I) — "not integrative" on the IRT and at a theoretically similar stage on one or both of the other tasks,
- *Transitional* (II) — either "integrative" or "not integrative" on the IRT but not at a theoretically similar stage on either of the other tasks, and
- *Primarily formal* (III) — "integrative" on the Selman IRT and at a theoretically similar stage on at least one of the other two tasks.

When necessary (and if possible) conservative backward extrapolations were used to estimate cognitive or pubertal status. The need for such a strategy arose if: (1) the onset of a depressive disorder occurred more than six months prior to the subject's entry into the study, (2) developmental staging data and clinical information could not be obtained within six months of each other after study entry, and (3) pertinent data were missing or incomplete. For backward extrapolations, we assumed that regression in either cognitive or pubertal stage cannot occur. Thus, if on the first available testing, the subject was at the lowest cognitive or somatosexual stage, it was presumed that had we tested the child at an earlier time, he or she would have been still at the lowest level of development. Backward extrapolation of pubertal status also used available pediatric norms (Buckler, 1979). For example, if, at intake, a ten-year-old girl in early puberty (Tanner II) had a depressive disorder that started when she was eight-and-a-half years old, then, according to the normative information, we could be 100 percent certain that she was prepubertal at the start of her depression.

Results

Developmental-Stage Characteristics of the Cohort at Intake. Table 1 depicts the developmental-stage distribution of the sample at study intake. The variable outcomes across the three cognitive tasks suggest that the measures do tap somewhat different capacities. In this regard, it is notable that reasoning in the interpersonal realm appeared to be the most difficult task for these depressed children; only 28 percent of them performed at the conceptually most abstract levels (levels III and IV).

The three-task index of cognitive development yielded a conser-

Table 1. Depressed Children's Developmental-Stage Distribution at Study Entry ($n = 80$)[a]

Measure	Cognitive-Developmental Stage				
	0	I	II	III	IV
Interpersonal reasoning task	4%	4%	64%	25%	3%
Combinations task		24%	20%	56%	
Personal identity interview		9%	42%	49%	
Three-task index		54%	26%	20%	

	Pubertal Stage	
	Prepubertal (I)	Pubertal (II-IV)
Pediatric examination according to Tanner (1962)	35%	65%

[a] Variable ns; some of the entries represent adjusted percents due to missing data.

vative stage-distribution relative to the outcomes on the individual measures (see Table 1). Table 1 also illustrates that the majority of the group had already entered puberty at the time of their enrollment in the study. This finding is consistent with the sample's chronological age spread.

The magnitude of the correlations among the three cognitive tasks underscores that it is sensible to use multiple measures to assess a developmental parameter. Performance on Mohr's PII correlated at $r = .41$, $p < .1110$ with each of the other two tasks. There was also a significant association between the Piagetian CT and Selman's IRT ($r = .26$, $p < .02$).

The relationship between chronological age and the two empirical indexes of development was in the expected direction. Namely, there was a significant, positive correlation between age and the global measure of cognitive stage ($r = .42$, $p < .0001$), and between age and pubertal status ($r = .67$, $p < .0001$). The association between pubertal status and cognitive stage was also significant ($r = .30$, $p < .01$).

Depressive Disorder Parameters and Developmental Stage. On the dimension of chronicity, the depressions that qualified a child for the study can be ranked as follows: adjustment disorder with depressed mood—most acute; major depressive disorder—intermediate; dysthymic disorder—most chronic. Data in support of this categorization have been reported (Kovacs and others, 1984a). Therefore, we examined our data to discover whether stage of development at the onset of the disorder predicted the eventual type of depression.

There was a negative association between cognitive stage at the onset of a disorder and the subsequent acuteness of the depression ($n = 61$, see Table 2). In other words, the children who were less cognitively mature at the onset of their depression were the most likely to have had a chronic disorder. Likewise, prepubertal onset predicted a more chronic depression ($n = 65$); age at onset was also inversely related to chronicity ($n = 80$, see Table 2).

As the data in Table 2 reveal, at the onset of the disorder the two developmental measures and age were also significantly intercorrelated. Therefore, the above analyses were repeated with the effect of the pertinent independent variable partialed out. When chronological age was statistically controlled, the relationship between cognitive stage and disorder chronicity dropped to nonsignificance; however, the association between pubertal status and disorder chronicity still remained (see Table 2). The partial correlation coefficients between age and depression type (with cognitive or pubertal stage held constant) further suggest that the association between the various developmental indexes and chronicity was due mostly to the effects of age and pubertal status.

The relationship between developmental stage at disorder onset and the length of time it took for individual children to recover from the depression was examined in cases with the diagnosis of major depressive

Table 2. Developmental Indexes at Onset of the Depressive Disorder and Its Subsequent Acuteness-Chronicity (Depression Type)[a]

	Correlation Coefficients			
	Depression type	Cognitive stage	Pubertal status	Age
Depression type	1.00			
Cognitive stage	−.21*	1.00		
Pubertal status	−.40***	.43***	1.00	
Age	−.27**	.52***	.81***	1.00

First-order partial correlation coefficients		Variable held constant
	Depression Type	
Cognitive stage	−.09	Age
Pubertal status	−.26*	Age
Age	−.19[b]	Cognitive stage
Age	.01	Pubertal status

[a] Variable ns.
[b] $p < .08$
*$p < .05$; **$p < .01$; ***$p < .001$

disorder. The statistical procedure was regression with incomplete survival data (Dixon and others, 1981), which provides an estimate of the association between the covariate and time-to-recovery (the criterion).

Pubertal status at disorder onset was negatively related to time-to-recovery from the major depression (Global χ^2 = 3.93, $p <$ .05, n = 38; regression coefficient = .87, S.E. = .451). In other words, prepubertal children had more prolonged episodes of major depression, whereas pubertal young people recovered more rapidly. However, cognitive stage at the onset of the major depression failed to predict time-to-recovery (Global χ^2 = 1.01, n.s., n = 48). Finally, the child's age when he or she developed the major depressive disorder was negatively related to time-to-recovery (Global, χ^2 = 8.49, $p <$ .005, n = 51; regression coefficient = .028, S.E. = .010).

Depressive Symptoms and Developmental Stage at Intake. The relationship between manifest symptoms and developmental stage was explored cross sectionally. The symptom data were the entire sample's child-interview based ratings from the intake ISCs, irrespective of the type of depressive disorder. Three analytical strategies were employed: (1) log-linear model analysis, (2) stepwise discriminant analysis, and (3) chi-square tests.

1. *Log-linear model analysis.* Based on the literature and our own assumptions, five triads of symptoms were used for hypothesis testing. Because of the requirements of log-linear analysis, the symptom ratings were dichotomized as "not present" (no or only minimal symptom severity) versus "present" (clinically significant rating). The operational cutoff scores for clinical significance on the various ISC symptom severity scales have been described elsewhere (Kovacs and others, 1984a).

- *Hypothesis 1:* "Pessimism/hopelessness, self-deprecation, and inability to experience pleasure are most likely to be associated with the formal stage rather than with the other two stages of cognitive development." The first model tested was the null hypothesis model of independence between presence or absence of the three symptoms and cognitive stage. According to the results, the null hypothesis could not be rejected (likelihood ratio $\chi^2(14)$ = 12.27, n.s.).
- *Hypothesis 2:* "Depressed mood and guilt are most likely to be associated with the formal stage, whereas feeling unloved and forlorn will be most evident at the other two cognitive stages." According to the results, the null hypothesis model of independence between the presence or absence of the above three symptoms and stage of cognitive development could not be rejected (likelihood ratio $\chi^2(12)$ = 11.21, n.s.).

- *Hypothesis 3:* "The three components of self-deprecation, namely, negative body image, negative view of one's abilities and talents, and worthlessness, are differentially mediated by cognitive stage." Because, in the development of self-identity, physical characteristics (as "me" attributes) emerge earlier than the more global "I" attributes (Damon and Hart, 1982), negative body image should predominate in the primarily concrete stage whereas worthlessness should be associated with the primarily formal stage.

The first model tested was the null hypothesis model of independence between the symptoms in question and the grouping variable. The null hypothesis was rejected (likelihood ratio $\chi^2(14) = 24.45$, $p < .04$). Then, a number of logical models were tested sequentially (for example, worthlessness is related to cognitive stage and the other two symptoms are independent of it). The simplest model that fit the observed data was one that involved an interaction of negative body image and perceived lack of ability with cognitive stage. A test of the latter model of interaction against the null hypothesis model of independence yielded a likelihood ratio of $\chi^2(6) = 13.20$, $p < .05$.

The distribution of the data revealed that negative body image and perceived lack of ability were independent of each other in the primarily concrete and primarily abstract stages but were strongly associated with one another in the transitional stage of cognitive development.

- *Hypothesis 4:* "Reduced sleep, decreased appetite, and fatigue are more likely to occur in conjunction with puberty than in the prepubertal stage." The null hypothesis model of independence between these three vegetative sysmptoms and pubertal status could not be rejected (likelihood ratio $\chi^2(7) = 13.68$, n.s.).
- *Hypothesis 5:* "Increased sleep, increased appetite, and excess energy are more likely to occur in prepuberty than puberty." Once again, the null hypothesis model of independence between the symptoms in question and pubertal status could not be rejected (likelihood ratio $\chi^2(6) = 4.54$, n.s.).

2. *Stepwise discriminant analyses.* As an alternate and potentially more sensitive test of the issues under consideration, two groups of ISC items (treated as continuous variables) were used to try to discriminate children at the various stages of development. One group of discriminating variables consisted of eight psychosocial symptoms including several that have been said to characterize "masked depression" in childhood (Glaser, 1968; Toolan, 1962); the other group of items encompassed six vegetative symptoms.

The first developmental parameter examined was stage of cognitive development. When the psychosocial symptoms were the discriminating variables, one canonical function was significant ($\chi^2(6) = 16.34$, $p < .01$). Three of the eight symptoms—anhedonia, disobedience, and somatic complaints—contributed to this significance. When the six vegetative symptoms were used to discriminate the three cognitive stages, one of the resultant canonical functions approached significance ($\chi^2(4) = 8.72$, $p < .07$).

Although the outcome of the former analysis was significant, only 57 percent of the known cases were correctly classified by the discriminant function. The classification matrix revealed that seventeen out of eighteen cases (94 percent) who tested at the transitional stage were grouped by the discriminant function into the primarily concrete stage. These results and the pertinent mean symptom ratings suggested that in the discriminant analysis the primarily concrete and the transitional cognitive stages were heuristically indistinct.

Therefore, the above analyses were repeated using a twofold cognitive stage schema: "not abstract" (primarily concrete or transitional) and "primarily abstract." The use of the eight psychosocial symptoms to discriminate this new dichotomous classification yielded a significant canonical function (see Table 3). The function correctly classified 87 percent of the cases with respect to cognitive stage. The excellent classification rate was accounted for mostly by the 100 percent accurate placement of the "not abstract" cases. As shown in Table 3, five symptoms were salient: compared to the "abstract" youngsters, the cognitively immature children ("not abstract") had higher levels of anhedonia and self-deprecation, but lower severity ratings on disobedience, somatic complaints, and pessimism.

Then, the six vegetative symptoms were used to try to discriminate the new twofold classification of cognitive development. However, the canonical function for these sets of variables did not reach statistical significance (see Table 3).

Pubertal status was the second developmental parameter examined. The set of eight psychosocial symptoms did discriminate between prepubertal and pubertal children (see Table 3). But only two of the eight symptoms—disobedience and anhedonia—were salient. As the standardized canonical discriminant function coefficients in Table 3 reveal, pubertal children had higher ratings on both variables than the prepubertal youth.

Notwithstanding the above findings, only 63 percent of the cases could be correctly classified with respect to somatosexual maturity. In

Table 3. Developmental Stage and Depressive Symptoms: Summary of the Results of Step-Wise Discriminant Function Analyses ($n = 80$)[a]

Grouping variable	Discriminating variable	Standardized discriminant function coefficient
	Psychosocial systems[b]	
Cognitive Stage	Pessimism	.35
	Guilt	—
	Self-deprecation	−.42
	Anhedonia	−.75
	Feeling unloved/forlorn	—
	Tantrums	—
	Somatic complaints	.40
	Disobedience	.62
	Vegetative symptoms[c]	
	Fatigue	—
	Excess energy	−.83
	Hypersomnia	—
	Hyposomnia	—
	Increased appetite	.68
	Decreased appetite	.55
	Psychosocial symptoms[d]	
Pubertal Stage	Pessimism	—
	Guilt	—
	Self-deprecation	—
	Anhedonia	.50
	Feeling unloved/forlorn	—
	Tantrums	—
	Somatic complaints	—
	Disobedience	.94
	Vegetative symptoms	
	Fatigue	
	Excess energy	None of the
	Hypersomnia	symptoms
	Hyposomnia	qualified for
	Increased appetite	the analysis
	Decreased appetite	

[a] ns are variable.
[b] Eigenvalue = .33, Canonical r = .50, Wilks' Lambda = .755, X^2 = 17.59 (5), $p < .004$.
[c] Eigenvalue = .11, Canonical r = .32, Wilks' Lambda = .897, X^2 = 6.91 (3), $p < .07$.
[d] Eigenvalue = .15, Canonical r = .36, Wilks' Lambda = .869, X^2 = 8.26 (2), $p < .02$.

addition, whereas the use of the psychosocial symptoms correctly classified 88 percent of the pubertal children, the rate of accuracy was only 10 percent for the cases whose pediatric scores placed them in prepuberty.

Finally, the analysis in which pubertal status was the grouping variable and in which the six vegetative symptoms were the discriminating variables failed to generate a canonical function. None of the symptoms satisfied the statistical criterion required for the analysis.

3. *Chi-square tests.* Because it has been generally presumed that young and immature children are far less likely to have thoughts of suicide than more mature children, the association between suicidal ideation and developmental stage was also examined. There was no relationship between stage of cognitive development and the children's reports of suicidal thoughts ($X^2(2) = 4.77$, n.s., $n = 70$). Likewise, prepubertal and pubertal youngsters were similarly likely to admit to having had ideas of killing themselves ($X^2(1) = 0.11$, n.s., $n = 68$).

Discussion

The field of developmental psychopathology brings together two domains: knowledge about the processes, mechanisms, and characteristics of development, and the vast clinical and empirical data about deviant behaviors (Rutter, in press). It reflects the belief that psychiatric disorders can be understood best within the matrix of the psychosocial and biological changes that characterize development (Elkind, 1982; Rutter, in press). Within this perspective, there are three important questions about the depressive disorders:

1. Are these disorders as common among children as among adults?
2. Are there age-related differences in the clinical symptom pictures?
3. What developmental processes and mechanisms can explain the differences that may exist (Rutter, in press)?

There have been few disagreements concerning the issue of prevalence. Although depression is one of the common psychiatric problems among adults (Secunda and others, 1973), its rarity in childhood has been observed clinically and has been verified by recent studies (Kashani and Simonds, 1979; Kashani and others, 1983; Makita, 1973; Poznanski and Zrull, 1970). As already noted, psychoanalytic as well as ego-analytic theory can provide explanations of the relatively low frequency of diagnosable depressive disorders in the preadult years. However, the rationale for the differential prevalence rates across the age span must be broader and more persuasive in order for it to be accepted by professionals of diverse theoretical persuasions.

The issue of age-related changes in the phenomenology of childhood depression has been far more controversial. The various clinical characterizations of the ways in which the disorder presumably manifests itself have led to confusion (Welner, 1978). Moreover, explanations of the putative changes in sumptomatology have been discordant and have lacked empirical support.

We believed, nonetheless, that a developmental approach to the depressions in childhood had merit and that some of the issues could be resolved by hypothesis testing and rigorous analytic procedures. Our sample was restricted to school-aged depressed youngsters because depressive disorders are difficult to diagnose unequivocally in preschoolers. We used longitudinal data on disorder characteristics and cross-sectional data on symptomatology in order to examine the role of development in the expression of depression. The pertinent literature suggested that it was sensible to select cognitive and pubertal development as the independent variables.

Notwithstanding our emphasis on methodological rigor, we were unable to verify even the most common notions about the developmental-stage mediation of depressive disorders in children. In fact, the findings were countertheoretical and counterintuitive. In our sample, the less mature children had the more chronic depressions; when in a major depressive episode, they also took far longer to recover than the more mature youth. Early age and prepubertal status at the onset of the depression were the two developmental markers that appeared to signal chronicity or prolonged recovery. Considered with the findings of Kovacs and others (1984a) that early onset is also associated with a more protracted dysthymic disorder in children, the present results highlight the salience of age with respect to outcome.

In regard to the relationship between developmental stage and depressive symptoms, the findings were inconsistent and, again, contrary to theoretical expectations. Whereas one analytic strategy—log-linear analysis—failed to reveal a meaningful symptomatic trend, another—stepwise discriminant analysis—indicated that the less mature children experienced the greatest disruption in hedonic capacity and the most self-denigration. And, in contrast to the literature, disobedient, oppositional behavior and complaints of aches and pains that presumably characterize the so-called masked depressions of younger children were far more evident among the cognitively and pubertally advanced youth.

Issues in the Assessment of Developmental Stage. The inability to confirm our hypotheses may be due, in part, to the complexity of the independent variable and the resultant measurement problem. The rationale for our three-task index of cognitive developmental stage has been already elucidated. Nonetheless, the manner in which we weighted the tasks and the appropriateness of the individual measures themselves are open to debate.

With respect to the former concern, it is worthwhile to note that, because the Piagetian tasks are the best standardized and the most widely used, we originally planned to employ the combinations task as the primary stage classifier. However, in view of the clinical syndrome under investigation, it was suggested to us that, of the three measures, the Selman task should carry the most weight. This suggestion was indirectly supported by the results of preliminary analyses. When the global stage of cognitive development was derived by assigning the greatest weight to the Piagetian task (as originally planned), the majority of the sample fell within the primarily formal classification. Such a cognitive-stage distribution did not make sense in light of the children's chronological age spread. Thus, the permutation of the tasks that was finally employed did appear to be the most sensible on clinical grounds and because it yielded a stage distribution that had better face validity.

With respect to the latter concern, it is indeed plausible that the measures themselves were not appropriate. However, it is unclear which other cognitive tasks could have better elucidated the relationship between developmental stage and the phenomenology of depression in the child. For example, Paulauskas (1983) used two measures of perspective taking to try to correlate the development of that cognitive capacity in children with their depressive symptoms. But she was also unable to verify her developmental theory-based hypotheses.

It could be contended further that our findings were confounded by the effect of psychopathology on general test performance. However, the depressed children performed in a variable fashion across the three cognitive measures. The latter result is similar to Selman's (1976) data on acting-out boys and argues against the likelihood that psychopathology produced a global inhibition or masking of cognitive capacities. Instead, it appears that our depressed subjects as well as Selman's (1976) behaviorally disturbed boys were delayed primarily in social reasoning. Therefore, compared to the emergence of other developmentally mediated potentials, a lag in the ability to think about and understand one's interpersonal world may be a marker of diagnosable child psychopathology. This interpretation appears to be consistent with reports that, among children, problems as diverse as attention deficit disorder or recently remitted major depression are associated with impaired peer relationships (Campbell and Paulauskas, 1979; Puig-Antich and Weston, 1983).

The Explanatory Power of Developmental Stage with Respect to the Expression of Depression. The expectation that less mature children have the briefest episodes of depression and the fastest recoveries can be predicated on egoanalytic theory (as already noted) and the documented biological resiliency that often characterizes the young. Based on the theory of Piaget (1950), it can be assumed further that only with the stage of formal operations does the child have the capacity to prolong the depression through ruminations about himself or herself and about his or her relationships to others. According to our data, however, cognitive stage appears to be unrelated to the duration or type of depression in the child. But early age or somatosexual immaturity at the onset of the disorder increases the likelihood of a serious bout of depression.

These findings have at least two explanations. First, it is possible that, as defined by age or pubertal stage, early onset reflects genetic or psychosocial vulnerability to depression or both. If that is the case, then early onset is merely a marker of risk, and it is the nature of the predisposing factors that must be elucidated.

Second, even in the absence of preexisting vulnerability, the relationship between early onset and the more serious and lengthy depressive disorders can be explained with reference to coping ability. The younger and less mature child probably lacks a sophisticated repertoire of internal coping responses and external coping resources that might help to resolve or ameliorate his or her distress. Thereby, the depression could become more prolonged.

Although stage of cognitive development had no explanatory power in our research with respect to characteristics of the depressive disorders, it did have some relevance to salient depressive symptoms. But, as already noted, the direction of the relationship was not generally in line with expectations. For example, the less mature child was as likely to have suicidal ideation as the cognitively more advanced youth. Therefore, the findings could imply that theories of cognitive, social-cognitive, and affective development derived and tested on normal children may have limited usefulness with respect to child psychopathology.

First, cognitive capacities or processes that are presumably necessary for the manifestation of certain symptoms may not be as critical as developmental theory would have it. For example, it has been generally assumed that because suicidal ideation implies a negation of one's own future, the symptom can occur only in the context of a full and elaborated sense of personal and historical time—that is, in adolescence or the stage of formal operations. Our results and the work of others (Carlson and Cantwell, 1982b) indicate that the former proposition is not a valid one.

In other words, symptomatic experience may not need to correspond to or be predicated on the existence of an underlying developmentally appropriate cognitive structure. Based on exposure to the media, role models (a depressed parent, for example), or older peers, a young school-aged child may learn semantic labels such as *suicide, depression,* or *hopelessness.* If the initial manifestations of depression are affective and somatic in nature, that is, disturbances in mood, hedonic capacity, and physical functions, the previously learned labels may serve to construe or verbalize the experience. Subsequently, the labels would be used appropriately in the context of the depression because they have taken on a personal meaning.

Another possible explanation of our findings concerning cognitive stage and symptom expression is that the functional significance of the prototypical progression of cognitive capacities is altered or obscured by early-onset psychopathology. If that is the case, then the available measures of cognitive developmental stage are inappropriate in the study of psychiatric disorders in juveniles.

Finally, it is notable that vegetative symptoms of depression did not follow a clear developmental pattern one way or another, and that we were unable to confirm their relationship to pubertal status. Because the relationship between biological maturation and psychopathological symptomatology has been a relatively unexplored area, the latter finding has no ready explanation.

Final Comments

The results obtained in our study suggest that the relationship between development, maturation, and the expression of depressive disorders among school-aged children is far more complicated than hitherto thought. The age- and stage-related features that were found strongly suggest that the study of developmental psychopathology may require new conceptual and explanatory strategies. But, in light of the mostly countertheoretical and counterintuitive findings, replications are clearly needed, as are tests and analyses on samples of preschool depressed children. Among younger probands, the developmental-stage mediation of disorder expression may be more in line with theoretical expectations.

References

American Psychiatric Association. *Diagnostic and Statistical Manual of Mental Disorders.* (3rd ed.) Washington, D.C.: American Psychiatric Association, 1980.

Beck, A. T. *Depression: Clinical, Experimental, and Theoretical Aspects.* New York: Hoeber, 1967.

Bemporad, J. "Manifest Symptomatology of Depression in Children and Adolescents." In S. Arieti and J. Bemporad (Eds.), *Severe and Mild Depression.* New York: Basic Books, 1978.

Bibring, E. "The Mechanism of Depression." In P. Greenacre (Ed.), *Affective Disorders.* New York: International Universities Press, 1953.

Buckler, J. M. H. *A Reference Manual of Growth and Development.* Oxford: Blackwell Scientific Publications, 1979.

Campbell, S. B., and Paulauskas, S. L. "Peer Relations in Hyperactive Children." *Journal of Child Psychology and Psychiatry,* 1979, *20,* 233-246.

Carlson, G. A., and Cantwell, D. P. "Unmasking Masked Depression in Children and Adolescents." *American Journal of Psychiatry,* 1980, *137* (4), 445-449.

Carlson, G. A., and Cantwell, D. P. "Diagnosis of Childhood Depression: A Comparison of the Weinberg and DSM-III Criteria." *Journal of the American Academy of Child Psychiatry,* 1982a, *21* (3), 247-250.

Carlson, G. A., and Cantwell, D. P. "Suicidal Behavior and Depression in Children and Adolescents." *Journal of the American Academy of Child Psychiatry,* 1982b, *21* (3), 361-368.

Conners, C. K. "Classification and Treatment of Childhood Depression and Depressive Equivalents." In D. M. Gallant and G. M. Simpson (Eds.), *Depression: Behavioral, Biochemical, Diagnostic and Treatment Concepts.* New York: Spectrum, 1976.

Cytryn, L., and McKnew, D. H. "Proposed Classification of Childhood Depression." *American Journal of Psychiatry,* 1972, *129* (2), 149-155.

Damon, W., and Hart, D. "The Development of Self-Understanding from Infancy through Adolescence." *Child Development,* 1982, *53,* 841-864.

Dixon, W. J., Brown, M. B., Engelman, L., Frane, J. W., Hill, M. A., Jennrich, R. I., and Toporek, J. D. (Eds.). *BMDP Statistical Software 1981.* Berkeley: University of California Press, 1981.

Elkind, D. "Piagetian Psychology and the Practice of Child Psychiatry." *Journal of the American Academy of Child Psychiatry,* 1982, *21* (5), 435-445.

Gaylin, W. (Ed.). *The Meaning of Despair: Psychoanalytic Contributions to the Understanding of Depression.* New York: Science House, 1968

Gelman, R. "Cognitive Development." *Annual Review of Psychology,* 1978, *29,* 297-332.

Glasberg, R., and Aboud, F. E. "A Developmental Perspective on the Study of Depression: Children's Evaluative Reactions to Sadness." *Developmental Psychology,* 1981, *17* (2), 195-202.

Glaser, K. "Masked Depression in Children and Adolescents." *Annual Progress in Child Psychiatry and Child Development,* 1968, *1,* 345-355.

Goodnow, J. J. "A Test of Milieu Effects with Some of Piaget's Tasks." *Psychological Monographs,* 1962, *76,* 1-21.

Herzog, D. B., and Rathbun, J. M. "Childhood Depression: Developmental Considerations." *American Journal of Diseases in Children,* 1982, *136,* 115-120.

Hollingshead, A. B. *Two Factor Index of Social Position.* Unpublished report. New Haven, Conn., 1957.

Jacobson, E. "Contribution to the Metapsychology of Cyclothymic Depression." In P. Greenacre (Ed.), *Affective Disorders.* New York: International Universities Press, 1953.

Kashani, J., and Simonds, J. F. "The Incidence of Depression in Children." *American Journal of Psychiatry,* 1979, *136* (9), 1203-1205.

Kashani, J. H., McGee, R. O., Clarkson, S. E., Anderson, J. C., Walton, L. A., Williams, S., Silva, P. A., Robins, A. J., Cytryn, L., and McKnew, D. H. "Depression in a Sample of Nine-Year-Old Children: Prevalence and Associated Characteristics." *Archives of General Psychiatry,* 1983, *40,* 1217-1223.

Kovacs, M. *Interview Schedule for Children: Form C and Follow-up Form.* Unpublished report. Pittsburgh, Pa., 1983.

Kovacs, M., and Beck, A. T. "An Empirical-Clinical Approach Toward a Definition of Childhood Depression." In J. G. Schulterbrandt and A. Raskin (Eds.), *Depression in Childhood: Diagnosis, Treatment and Conceptual Models.* New York: Raven Press, 1977.

Kovacs, M., Feinberg, T. L., Crouse-Novak, M. A., Paulauskas, S. L., and Finkelstein, R. "Depressive Disorders in Childhood: I. A Longitudinal Prospective Study of Characteristics and Recovery." *Archives of General Psychiatry,* 1984a, *41,* 229-237.

Kovacs, M., Feinberg, T. L., Crouse-Novak, M. A., Paulauskas, S. L., Pollock, M., and Finkelstein, R. "Depressive Disorders in Childhood: II. A Longitudinal Study of the Risk for a Subsequent Major Depression." *Archives of General Psychiatry,* 1984b, *41,* 643-649.

Lefkowitz, M. M., and Burton, N. "Childhood Depression: A Critique of the Concept." *Psychological Bulletin,* 1978, *85* (4), 716-726.

Makita, K. "The Rarity of 'Depression' in Childhood." *Acta Paedopsychiatrica,* 1973, *40,* 37-44.

Malmquist, C. P. "Major Depression in Childhood: Why Don't We Know More?" *American Journal of Orthopsychiatry,* 1983, *53* (2), 262-268.

McConville, B. J., Boag, L. C., and Purohit, A. P. "Three Types of Childhood Depression." *Canadian Psychiatric Association Journal,* 1973, *18,* 133-138.

Mohr, D. M. "Development of Attributes of Personal Identity." *Developmental Psychology,* 1978, *14,* 427-428.

Paulauskas, S. L. "A Cognitive-Developmental Analysis of Self-Image Disparity in Depressed Children." Unpublished doctoral dissertation, University of Pittsburgh, 1983.

Piaget, J. *The Psychology of Intelligence.* New York: Harcourt Brace, 1950.

Piaget, J., and Inhelder, B. *The Origin of the Idea of Chance in Children.* New York: W. W. Norton, 1975.

Poznanski, E., and Zrull, J. P. "Childhood Depression: Clinical Characteristics of Overtly Depressed Children." *Archives of General Psychiatry,* 1970, *23,* 8-15.

Preskorn, S. H., Weller, E. B., and Weller, R. A. "Depression in Children: Relationship Between Plasma Imipramine Levels and Response." *Journal of Clinical Psychiatry,* 1982, *43* (11), 450-453.

Puig-Antich, J., and Weston, B. "The Diagnosis and Treatment of Major Depressive Disorder in Childhood." *Annual Review of Medicine,* 1983, *34,* 231-245.

Puig-Antich, J., Blau, S., Marx, N., Greenhill, L. L., and Chambers, W. "Prepubertal Major Depressive Disorder: A Pilot Study." *Journal of the American Academy of Child Psychiatry,* 1978, *17* (4), 695-707.

Puig-Antich, J., Chambers, W., Halpern, F., Hanlon, C., and Sachar, E. J. "Cortisol Hypersecretion in Prepubertal Depressive Illness: A Preliminary Report." *Psychoneuroendocrinology,* 1979, *4,* 191-197.

Puig-Antich, J., Goetz, R., Hanlon, C., Davies, M., Thompson, J., Chambers, W. J., Tabrizi, M. A., and Weitzman, E. D. "Sleep Architecture and REM Sleep Measures in Prepubertal Children with Major Depression: A Controlled Study." *Archives of General Psychiatry,* 1982, *39,* 932-939.

Rie, H. E. "Depression in Childhood: A Survey of Some Pertinent Contributions." *Journal of the American Academy of Child Psychiatry,* 1966, *5,* 653-685.

Rochlin, G. "The Loss Complex: A Contribution to the Etiology of Depression." *Journal of the American Psychoanalytic Association,* 1959, *7,* 299-316.

Rubin, K. H. "Egocentrism in Childhood: A Unitary Construct?" *Child Development,* 1973, *44,* 102-110.

Rubin, K. H. "Role Taking in Childhood: Some Methodological Considerations." *Child Development,* 1978, *49,* 428-433.

Rutter, M. "The Developmental Psychopathology of Depression: Issues and Perspectives." In M. Rutter, C. Izard, and P. Read (Eds.), *Depression: Developmental Perspectives.* New York: Guilford, in press.

Schwartz, R. M., and Trabasso, T. "Children's Understanding of Emotions." In C. E. Izard, J. Kagan, and R. Zajonc (Eds.), *Emotions, Cognition, and Behavior.* New York: Cambridge University Press, in press.

Secunda, S. K., Katz, M. M., Friedman, R. J., and Schuyler, D. *The Depressive Disorders.* Department of Health, Education and Welfare Publication No. (HSM) 73-9157. Washington, D.C.: U.S. Government Printing Office, 1973.

Selman, R. L. "Toward a Structural Analysis of Developing Interpersonal Relations Concepts: Research with Normal and Disturbed Preadolescent Boys." In A. Pick (Ed.), *Tenth Annual Minnesota Symposium on Child Psychology.* Minneapolis: University of Minnesota Press, 1976.

Selman, R. L. *The Growth of Interpersonal Understanding: Developmental and Clinical Analyses.* New York: Academic Press, 1980.

Selman, R. L., Jaquette, D., and Bruss-Saunders, E. *Assessing Interpersonal Understanding: An Interview and Scoring Manual in Five Parts.* Unpublished manuscript. Cambridge, Mass., 1979.

Shantz, C. U. "The Development of Social Cognition." In E. M. Hetherington (Ed.), *Review of Child Development Research.* Vol. 5. Chicago: University of Chicago Press, 1975.

Siomopoulos, G., and Inamdar, S. C. "Developmental Aspects of Hopelessness." *Adolescence,* 1979, *14* (53), 233-239.

Spitzer, R. L., Endicott, J., and Robins, E. "Research Diagnostic Criteria: Rationale and Reliability." *Archives of General Psychiatry,* 1978, *35,* 773-782.

Tanner, J. M. *Growth at Adolescence.* (2nd ed.) Oxford: Blackwell Scientific, 1962.

Toolan, J. M. "Depression in Children and Adolescents." *American Journal of Orthopsychiatry,* 1962, *32,* 404-414.

Welner, Z. "Childhood Depression: An Overview." *Journal of Nervous and Mental Disease,* 1978, *166* (8), 588-593.

Wessman, A. E., and Gorman, B. S. "The Emergence of Human Awareness and Concepts of Time." In B. S. Gorman, and A. E. Wessman (Eds.), *The Personal Experience of Time.* New York: Plenum, 1977.

Maria Kovacs is an associate professor of psychiatry at the University of Pittsburgh School of Medicine, Department of Psychiatry, and director of the Childhood Depression Research Program at the Western Psychiatric Institute and Clinic.

Stana L. Paulauskas is a research associate at the University of Pittsburgh School of Medicine, Department of Psychiatry, and coordinator of the Childhood Depression Project at the Western Psychiatric Institute and Clinic.

Studies of offspring of depressed parents are reviewed. A program of research on young children of unipolar and bipolar depressed parents is described. Early manifestations or precursors of childhood depression are identified.

Young Offspring of Depressed Parents: A Population at Risk for Affective Problems

Carolyn Zahn-Waxler, E. Mark Cummings
Ronald J. Iannotti, Marian Radke-Yarrow

It is such a secret place, this land of tears.
de Saint Exupéry, 1943

The purpose of this chapter is to use principles from the emerging domain of developmental psychopathology in order to study possible early manifestations, precursors, or prototypes of childhood depression. In developmental psychopathology the focus is on the multiple processes and pathways by which early patterns of individual adaptation evolve to later patterns of adaptation (Sroufe and Rutter, 1984; Rutter and Garmezy, 1984). The aim is to understand the contributions of biology and experience to the origins and course of disordered behavior, whether disorder emerges in earliest childhood or not until adulthood.

This chapter, written by employees of the U.S. government, is considered to be in the public domain and thus is not eligible for copyright.
We are deeply appreciative of the help from Rita Dettmers in the preparation of the manuscript.

Implicit in the developmental model is the necessity of obtaining developmental data on both normal and deviant functioning (Cicchetti, 1984). Thus, longitudinal and age cross-sectional research designs are important features of this approach. Overarching goals of developmental psychology include: (1) the development of more comprehensive theories of the etiology of emotional problems, and (2) the collection of information that may be used to establish effective intervention and prevention strategies. The research reported in this chapter focuses on a little-explored area within the field—factors contributing to individual differences in social functioning, emotional expression, and emotional modulation in children during the first years of life. Ultimately the researchers hope to identify response patterns that evolve into diagnosable affective disturbance.

The Study of Depression

Etiology of Depression. Many theories have been used to explain the etiology of depression in both children and adults (see Akiskal and McKinney, 1975; Kashani and others, 1981; and Rutter and Garmezy, 1984). Most explanations are based on variants of psychoanalytic, social learning, cognitive, genetic, or biochemical theories. Because many hypotheses ascribe the origins of adult depression to childhood determinants, there tends to be considerable continuity between explanations of childhood and adult depression. This overlap in emphasis suggests the usefulness of an explicitly developmental psychopathological research perspective: Adoption of such an approach would permit direct, prospective investigation of (1) antecedents and correlates of childhood depression and (2) factors in childhood that produce later depression.

Among the major variables hypothetically associated with the development of depression are the following:
1. absence or loss of mother or other persons significant in the life of the child (Bibring, 1953; Bowlby, 1980);
2. the development of insecure attachments to parents, and, hence, the development of fragile, tenuous social relationships with others outside the family setting as well;
3. failure to develop autonomy as a consequence of inadequate development of self-concept and self-esteem (Miller, 1981);
4. exposure to atypical childrearing practices, including a range of parental factors that might make the child feel sad, helpless, confused, or self-deprecatory—for example, inconsistent parental behavior (Anthony, 1975; Davenport and

others, 1979), emotional unavailability (Emde, 1980), parental derision, failure to nurture, and rejection (Crook and others, 1981);

5. development of learned helplessness or depressogenic cognitive and attributional styles, which result from exposure to inescapable, uncontrollable aversive experiences (Beck, 1979; Seligman and Maier, 1967);
6. loss of (or inability to use) social supports in times of stress and distress (Davenport and others, 1979); and
7. biological vulnerability or genetic predisposition toward affective illness (see review by Meyersberg and Post, 1979).

There is overlap in these different emphases and different factors may work in combination to produce affective disturbance. Temperament, personality, familial factors, sociodemographic characteristics, neurobiological disturbances, life situations, and stress all may play etiologic roles in the development of depressive illness. In our research we have emphasized the importance of yet another set of conditions that may place children at risk for depression: Chronic exposure to a depressed person's moods and emotional dysregulation may itself create a climate for depression, with (empathic) contagion of negative emotions being a process by which depression is transmitted.

The utility of the different theories can ultimately be determined only by research that systematically investigates the etiologic role of these different factors during the course of development. One step in this process is to discover when depression begins and what are its early manifestations and precursor patterns in the formative stages of development (Zahn-Waxler and others, 1984a; Stern, 1983; Provence, 1983). The early work of Spitz (1946) on anaclitic depression in infancy and the work of Gaensbauer and Hiatt (1984), who recently identified depression in a three-month-old infant, suggest very early origins of depression. But most assessment procedures do not achieve sufficient accuracy for formally diagnosing depression until the child is five to six years old and able to introspect, to a degree, about internal affective stages. Many theories, as well, would predict that the child would have to be at least latency age and have perspective on past and future events in order for adultlike depression to occur. Alternative research strategies are needed to address these issues. Approaches are required that identify a sample of children at risk for affective disturbance and that use observational and experimental procedures capable of uncovering a wide range of socioemotional functioning, since early manifestations of depression in young children may not necessarily fit the classic signs.

Research Strategies. A number of research strategies have been used to study childhood depression. Psychoanalytic approaches have favored retrospective accounts by patients and the cumulative wisdom and penetrating insights of the clinician as the major data source (for example, Miller, 1981). A second approach has been to begin directly with the depressed child and to study current functioning, employing structured interviews, observational procedures and biochemical assays (for example, Kovacs, this volume; Poznanski and others, 1982; Puig-Antich, 1982). Still another approach has been to study children at risk for depression by investigating their functioning in relation to biological, constitutional, and environmental risk factors that might predispose them toward affective illness. Recently, a number of studies have focused on children with an affectively ill parent, the assumption being that these children would be particularly at risk for depression (see review by Beardslee and others, 1983). This is the approach we have used to sample and study signs of depression in very young children.

Offspring (High-Risk) Studies. A series of studies of offspring of depressed parents have, indeed, suggested that children of parents with diagnosed affective disorders appear to comprise a group at risk for the development of depressive disorders (for example, see review by Orvaschel and others, 1980). The number of studies is few and methodological problems characterize much of the research. Many of the family studies have been retrospective and the data may have been biased or influenced by the proband's illness. Recently, however, there has been an increase in prospective studies of offspring of depressed parents. A major issue addressed in these studies is the degree of concordance of diagnosis in parent and child. Some of the investigators, however, examine a wider range of psychosocial, affective, and cognitive functioning (in parent and/or child) than can be obtained by diagnosis alone (for example, Goodman, 1983; Hammon and Hiroto, 1983; Hops and others, 1983; Radke-Yarrow and others, 1982; Musick and others, 1983). This extension of investigation to variables beyond those symptoms used to diagnose depression becomes particularly important in developmental studies: Signs and symptoms of depression may differ at different ages, and if the measurement net is cast too narrowly, significant predictor variables will be missed.

In earlier studies of children of schizophrenic parents, cognitive, perceptual, and memory functions were the primary outcome variables that were assessed in the offspring because of their logical connection to problems experienced by adult schizophrenics. Children of depressed parents often were used as one type of control group in these studies and hence, initially, there was more information available about cognitive/perceptual than socioemotional behavior in those offspring. However, disturbances in socioemotional functioning would be presumed to be more reflective of problems related to depression. A few of these offspring studies did examine indexes of socioemotional and interpersonal functioning in older children with a depressed parent. Those studies provide some clues about socioemotional variables that might profitably be studied in younger children as precursor variables. Rolf (1976) and Weintraub and others (1978) have studied the peer relationships and school behavior of children with normal, depressed, and schizophrenic parents. Weintraub and others (1978) have reported that children of depressed as well as schizophrenic mothers were rated by teachers and peers as more disturbed than children of normal controls on measures of impatience, defiance, withdrawal, disturbed classroom behavior, aggression, and unhappiness. Another group of investigators studied adolescents whose mothers had been psychotic during the child's infancy (Grunebaum and others, 1978; Kauffman and others, 1979). They, too, reported significantly less social competence in children with depressed mothers than in those with mothers with nonaffective diagnoses. Whether children with less severely impaired, but nonetheless depressed, parents, would show parallel problems is currently unknown. There is also a need to study the question of whether the same children who show certain manifestations of emotional disturbance will later show depression.

The major goal of offspring research is to study patterns in intergenerational transmission of affective disorder and to establish the conditions that contribute to concordance and discordance in problems of parents and children. Ultimately, as noted earlier, it will be necessary to identify the specific biological and experiential factors that contribute to the development of depression (or related problems) in the offspring whether the difficulties occur when they are still children, or are manifested later, in adolescence or adulthood. There are many intervening steps in the research process between initial descriptive statements and final identification of such causal influences.

Precursor Studies. Our beginning research strategy has been, first, to try to describe some of the social and emotional problems very young children of depressed parents encounter and manifest, and then to discover which of the problems or areas of concern might eventually culminate in diagnosable depressive disorders. We have attempted to characterize the emotions the children are exposed to in the home environment and to discuss how these might be associated with particular problematic child behaviors. Global measures of emotions in the home were used: for example, type of diagnosed parental depression, prevailing mood as reported by the parent, quality of maternal functioning observed in the home, and mothers' reports of childrearing values, attitudes, and philosophies. In a more speculative vein, we have also sought to establish the nature of caregivers' own social and emotional relationships. Another component of this research has been to construct experimental affective environments in the laboratory that are sometimes pleasurable and sometimes challenging. Individual differences in children's patterns of social and emotional responses are then explored. First, we give a description of initial work on two-year-old children with a manic-depressive parent, followed by a description of findings from a parallel study of children with a unipolar depressed parent. We then briefly consider longitudinal follow-up work in progress on these samples of children (now five to six years old) in which we are examining continuity of affective styles and coping strategies under experimental conditions. The goal of this longitudinal approach is to understand better why some children at risk are able to cope adequately while other children evidence emotional problems and depressive symptomatology.

Study One: Children of Bipolar Parents

In bipolar illness, episodes of mania as well as depression occur. Mania is expressed through hyperactivity, overtalkativeness, flight of ideas, inflated self-esteem or grandiosity, and risk taking. Irritability and hostility are not uncommon accompaniments and high levels of conflict between manic-depressives and their spouses have been reported. There is considerable variability in both frequency and severity of expression of manic symptoms. Current theories emphasize the biological underpinnings of bipolar illness. Lithium carbonate helps regulate the mood swings and is typically the treatment of choice. Bipolar illness has been reported to aggregate in families (for example, Davenport and others, 1979). Latency-aged children and adolescents with a bipolar parent have been reported to be at increased risk for depression (Cytryn and others, 1982), and to show other symptoms as well, such as anxiety, sleep problems, and isolating behavior (for example, Mayo and others, 1979). Both genetic (for example, Fieve and others, 1973) and environmental mechanisms for intergenerational transmission of bipolar illness have been suggested. Investigating emotional problems close to their points of origin through direct observational study of very young children might help to clarify the types of causal questions ultimately to be addressed.

The major symptoms of depression include disregulation of emotions (for example, excessive or inappropriate expression of sadness, guilt, lack of pleasure) and withdrawal from social relations.

Mania produces still further disregulation, disorganization, and unpredictability in interpersonal relations: We expected its influence on children to be particularly strong. Davenport and others (1979) present the hypothesis that there are enduring interpersonal psychodynamics characteristic of bipolar families that may help to perpetuate bipolar illness across generations. These include (1) difficulties in initiating and sustaining intimacy apart from the family; (2) difficulties in mastering issues of loss, grief, and rage; and (3) development of defensive maneuvers in order to avoid confrontation with conflict. Anthony (1975), too, described chronic deficiencies in bipolar adults that could create problems in parenting and could put the developing child at risk, for example: (1) taking but refusing to give, (2) having little awareness of others as people and hence little ability to empathize, and (3) having diminished capacity for forging stable, affectional bonds with the child. Children's socioemotional development in parallel areas of functioning would appear to provide especially fruitful areas of inquiry: Because problems with empathy, affection, and conflict resolution could create enduring difficulties and hence perpetuate bipolar symptoms, it is logical to look at the course of their development, prospectively, beginning early in childhood. Whether or not disturbances in these areas are unique to bipolar illness or characterize other forms of psychopathology as well, is still an open issue.

To assess children's functioning, we created experimental analogues of affective environments intended to elicit a range of socioemotional behaviors. The experimental conditions were designed to represent challenges, joys, and difficulties encountered, to a certain degree, in the lives of all children. The conditions simultaneously were intended to represent potential problem areas in families with an affectively ill parent. We reasoned that children from such families would be predisposed to be reactive to situations that most children could take in stride. Specifically, the experimental manipulations were designed to make it possible to examine how children (1) explored a new social environment; (2) dealt with sorrow and distress in others; (3) coped with stressful background events (for example, conflicts or arguments between others); (4) handled separation from the caregiver; and (5) dealt with imposed frustrations.

Measures of children's functioning included their friendly, social interactions; altruistic or prosocial behaviors; aggressive behaviors or propensities for conflict; and expression and regulation of positive and negative emotions in the context of ongoing social interactions. We tried to incorporate into our assessments dimensions of socioemotional functioning that could be directly tied to depressive symptoms (for example, distress, social withdrawal) and also closely related dimensions that might be more appropriately conceptualized as indexes of social competence and social problem-solving strategies (Spivack and Shure, 1974; Weintraub and others, 1978). For example, we devised codes for commonly defined components of social competence including behavioral categories such as threaten, share, cooperate, and avoid and affective dimensions such as impatience, emotionality, and aggression. The primary data reported in this chapter are based on the child's functioning, principally outside the family setting. If problems were beginning, our method of study allowed us to see to what degree difficulties had generalized to affect the child in his or her extrafamilial world. We also assessed prosocial behavior of the caregiver, since clinicans have observed a tendency for the early assumption of a caregiver role in children from families where parents are highly distressed (for example, Miller, 1981).

Sample. Seven males with bipolar parents were studied longitudinally beginning at age one. The families previously had been treated as inpatients or outpatients at the National Institute of Mental Health and had been part of a biomedical research project on bipolar illness. All but one had been treated with lithium. No parents were hospitalized during the course of the study and technically all were in remission at the time of the study. The Schedule of Affective Disorders and Schizophrenia–Lifetime Version (SADS-L) diagnostic interview and DSM-III (American Psychiatric Association, 1980) criteria also were used to confirm diagnoses of history of bipolar illness. In four of the families the mother had been the ill parent; in the remaining three families it was the father. The seven offspring were compared with a group of twenty children (ten boys and ten girls) of parents without serious current affective disorders. Extensive but unsuccessful recruitment efforts had been expended to obtain a sample of one-year-old females from bipolar families. Proband and control groups were matched on relevant demographic characteristics. Procedures and results are summarized below. (See Zahn-Waxler and others, 1984a, for more extended discussion of sampling and other issues of reliability, validity, methodology, statistics, and results.)

Home Assessments. The children of bipolar parents and the control group were studied primarily in home settings. Cognitive, neurological, physical, and socioemotional functioning and parent-child interactions were assessed. Staff visits were made by the same home visitor on a monthly basis. Every other month, testers (some of whom were blind to parent diagnosis) visited the home. At the end of the year, home visitors provided summary assessments of problem behaviors in the children. Some of these measures provided preliminary signs of early problem behaviors in children of bipolar parents (Zahn-Waxler and others, 1984b).

One child was reported to show severe depression, manifested in apathy, flat affect, sadness, serious difficulties in relating to others and in regulating of affect, and a marked tendency to fall asleep when exposed to new or stressful stimulation. He was referred, along with his manic-depressive mother, for treatment. Another child's patterns of attachment and development of individuation were so inappropriate and undifferentiated that he cried frequently at the departure of the home visitor, called strangers "Mom," and called others by his own first name. A third child was identified as highly aggressive and a fourth child had considerable difficulty relating to others, being described as "cold," "flat," and "spooky" by outside observers. Yet another child showed disregulation of emotion, intense and unusual phobias, and general emotional immaturity. It must be noted, however, that these assessments were made by persons knowledgeable about the parental diagnoses, and parents had considerable input into reports of children's symptoms.

Standardized assessment procedures were used to see if problem behaviors would be observed in children's cognitive and socioemotional functioning when observers were uninformed about the parental diagnoses. On cognitive tests of physical object permanence of visual self-recognition, children from bipolar families did not show impairments. On tasks that involved interpersonal relations or social problem-solving abilities, children with a bipolar parent showed significant deficits (Zahn-Waxler and others, 1982): These children had less secure attachments (assessed using a modified strange situation) and more problems in rudimentary role-taking abilities (assessed using the agent-use task of Watson and Fischer, 1977) than had controls.

Laboratory Assessments. When children reached the age of two, they came for laboratory assessments on three occasions, the first two of which are reported on here. The purpose was to see whether early signs of difficulty were real and enduring and whether they had generalized to social relations with others outside the family setting. In each session, children were observed with a different familiar playmate of the same age. Interactions with an unfamiliar adult were also examined. Sessions were videotaped and data were coded from videotapes by pairs of observers uninformed of parental diagnoses.

Each of the two sessions began with the child interacting with his or her playmate in an apartment-like setting with the mothers nearby. Their behaviors were observed under a range of conditions variously conducive to enjoyment, conflict, distress, or frustration. These conditions included:

1. *A novel environment.* Children's initial play in a new room and situation (five minutes).
2. *A background climate of affection and sharing.* Two female adults entered the adjoining kitchen. They greeted the mothers and children, then cooperated with each in a warm, friendly fashion while getting refreshments for the mothers and children (five minutes).
3. *A neutral context.* There were no experimental interventions (five minutes).
4. *A background climate of hostility, anger, and rejection.* The women returned and had a verbal argument while washing the dishes. Each angrily accused the other of not doing her share of work around the building (five minutes).
5. *A second neutral context* (five minutes).
6. *A reconciliation* in which the adults returned, greeted each other with affection, and apologized for their unpleasant behavior (2 minutes).
7. *A friend's separation experience.* The mother of the proband child's friend was asked to leave the room (1 minute).
8. *Separation from mother.* The proband's own mother was called from the room as well (1 minute).
9. *Reunion with mother.* Both mothers returned (4 minutes).

The following responses were coded during each of the periods described above:

- *Interpersonal physical aggression* — acts of hitting, kicking, pushing, or throwing things;
- *object struggles* — attempts to grab or take another's possession;
- *undirected aggression* — aggression against the physical environment, for example, throwing things against the floor, kicking toys;
- *intense aggression* — aggression that was violent or potentially dangerous;
- *Passivity* — no response or crying only in the face of aggression;
- *altruism or prosocial behavior* — help, cooperation, sharing, providing comfort or sympathy, or aid in a noninterpersonal mode (such as cleaning up);
- *social interactions* — friendly, interactive play such as invitations to join in an ongoing activity, games of chase, and so on; and
- *emotional expressiveness* — coded as *positive affect, anger, distress,* and total *emotionality.*

Structured situations also were used to assess children's emotionality, sociability, aggression, and altruism outside the peer relationship. A mildly frustrating situation was initiated by an unfamiliar female adult who took a toy away from the child. Simulations of distress (pain and sadness) by the mother and female experimenter, and a taped cry of an infant were also used as stimuli for empathy and altruism. These events occurred over the course of the sessions, each of which was one and one-half hours in length, and were interwoven in a natural way into ongoing play and learning situations. Responses coded during the structured situations with adults were as follows: Behavioral reactions toward the adult following frustration were scored for *persistence* and *intensity of physical aggression* or struggles for control over the toy. Prosocial behaviors and other patterns of coping with distress included the following: *altruism* (help, sharing, comfort, and cooperation); *caregiver role* indicating internalization of responsibility (inferred from adultlike mannerisms or unusually skillful, competent prosocial acts); *prolonged orientation to distress* (diminished ability to withdraw from other's distress and re-engage in other activities); *emotional concern* (facial or vocal expressions of concern, indicating empathy or worry); *seeking information, guidance,* or *reassurance* from mother. Dimensions of emotionality coded during peer interactions also were coded here. Scores were summed across sessions for statistical analyses.

Results. Children from bipolar families showed patterns of functioning that continued to differ from those of children from control families. These two-year-old children's interactions and relationships with others outside the family setting and their capacities for emotion regulation appeared to be undermined by the imposition of challenging, sometimes stressful, conditions. This generalization is based on multiple statistical analyses in which the seven proband children were compared with the twenty controls. Boys and girls in the control group were combined for analysis after it was determined that they did not differ significantly along sexual lines. In the findings detailed below, significance levels for reported differences typically are $p < .05$ or better.

Antisocial Behavior/Aggression. There were strong group differences in aggression toward the unfamiliar adult: Children from bipolar families were more intense and persistent in their aggression; they fought harder and longer to retrieve the object that the adult had taken from them. Children from the two groups did not differ on overall levels of aggression toward playmates, or on the specific components of aggression such as physical attacks or object conflicts. Children from bipolar homes did show more undirected aggression than controls. And in one situation—experimentally imposed separation from mother— children from bipolar families tended to show intense aggression to their playmates. Following their mothers' return these children were more likely to show intense (displaced) aggression toward their playmates. Finally, when aggressed against, children from bipolar families were somewhat less likely to fight back. Under certain, sometimes stressful, conditions, then, these children appeared to have less mature, direct, or adaptive methods of dealing with conflict.

Prosocial Behavior/Altruism. A majority of the children responded altruistically when the mother simulated distress, extremely few responded to the experimenter's simulated distress, and about one-third of them made prosocial efforts with regard to the infant. There were no differences between children from bipolar and control families during any of these distress simulations on any of the specific measures of altruism. Children from bipolar homes, however, showed more preoccupation with simulations of pain and sadness. They were less able to withdraw from the distress and re-engage in other activities. Further, they had more difficulty using their mothers as sources of reassurance and guidance during the experimenter and infant simulations than controls. Problems in prosocial functioning in children with an affectively ill parent were more apparent in children's relationships with their playmates. Children with a bipolar parent showed less frequent altruism toward their peers than controls during ongoing play activities, which was reflected specifically in less sharing and somewhat helping.

Emotional Expressiveness and Social Interactions During Peer Play. Analysis of friendly, social interactions indicated that children from bipolar families engaged in less social interaction than controls in all of the play sessions. Different patterns of emotionality induced by the environmental challenges appeared to accompany the different patterns of sociability. During peer play, children from bipolar families (relative to controls) showed high levels of distress during the simulated argument, and low levels of pleasure immediately following the conflict.

Discussion. As a group, children from bipolar families appeared to have more than their share of socioemotional difficulties and to lack competence in their interpersonal relations. The experimentally manipulated conditions of separation, suffering, and hostility had the effect of highlighting group differences in children's emerging abilities to regulate emotion and engage in social relationships with others. The sometimes inappropriate timing of their aggression may have made them appear more aggressive, even though they were not particularly aggressive most of the time. Their difficulty in sharing and socializing with agemates also may be indicative of the early establishment of barriers to adaptive functioning in their own social worlds. These early social deficits may represent precursors to later diagnosable affective disturbance, perhaps to depression.

There is reason to hypothesize that these interpersonal difficulties are mediated, in part, by poor modulation of affect. In many different circumstances, children with a bipolar parent showed greater reactivity than controls following the introduction of psychological stressors. We recorded, for example, heightened upset during others' fights, preoccupation with others' pain and sorrow, and intense displaced aggression following separation from the mother.

There are caveats to the conclusions drawn from this research. The study was based on a very small number of index cases, all of whom are males. The sex of the bipolar parent varied but most of the assessments were obtained through the mother, because the bipolar fathers were not ready participants in the research. Most of the bipolar parents had spouses with unipolar depression, so the child sometimes was exposed to multiple and different forms of depression, ranging in degree of severity. Hence, the degree to which these findings are psychopathology-specific cannot be ascertained here. With these warnings, we provide further data on the emotional climate to which these children were exposed and consider their possible implications for socioemotional development.

Data from the mothers, who had been asked to report systematically on their moods, indicated differences in mothers from bipolar and control families. The former reported more sadness, fear, rage, and anhedonia than the latter (Zahn-Waxler and others, 1984b). Observations by home visitors of mothers' functioning also yielded differences. Mothers from bipolar homes were viewed as somewhat more disorganized, ineffective, and inconsistent in their caregiving. They also looked sadder and more tense, and were more lacking in energy (Davenport and others, 1984).

On a childrearing practices Q-sort (Block, 1965), which indicates values, attitudes, and philosophies about childrearing, mothers from the two groups differed, not so much on issues having to do with teaching and discipline as on clusters of items having to do with issues surrounding expression of emotion. Mothers from bipolar families were less likely than controls to encourage the child to be open to new experience, less likely to be open in their own expression of emotion, more likely to be protective of the child and to teach the child to control feelings, and more likely to have negative affect toward the child (Davenport and others, 1984). It is reasonable to assume that such attitudes and values, if actually conveyed in the parent's behavior and experienced by the child, could have significant implications for the child's socioemotional development from very early childhood. The findings are consistent with clinical reports in which such families explicitly emphasize the need to contain and suppress emotions because of the chronic fear of emotional explosions (that is, the manic episodes). If attempts at suppression of affect generalize to interactions with the children, they could, ironically, help contribute to the very disregulation that might place some of these children at later risk for bipolar depression. This is just one of many sets of stressful circumstances that might be expected to converge on children who have a seriously affectively ill parent.

The children of manic-depressives do appear, even at an early age, to be overly reactive to externally imposed stressors and to recover slowly, even after the noxious stimulation has been removed. This could reflect early forerunners of learned helplessness. The reasons for disregulation of affect and heightened sensitivity to stress may lie in the biology of the individual children, various features of the environments in which they are reared (such as chronic exposure to high levels of negative emotion), or both. Exposure to environmental stressors has been shown to result in a number of biological changes in organisms: for example, changes in brain structure (Kandell, 1982), changes in the immune system (Gross and Siegel, 1982), and changes in brain opioid systems (Pansepp, in press). Meyersberg and Post (1979) have demonstrated that an organism who has become sensitized by repeated exposure to externally imposed noxious stimulation (for example, to shock), will later respond (for example, with epileptic seizures) to smaller doses of shock than initially required to elicit a seizure. Reasoning by analogy, Meyersberg and Post (1979) have discussed ways in which aversive psychological stimulation might operate similarly. In the case of children from affectively disturbed families, it may take relatively little emotional disturbance in the environment to trigger distress and affect disregulation, because of these children's greater than normal early exposure to negative emotions. Thus, there may be compelling historical, environmental bases for apparent "overreaction" to stress.

Our research design does not make it possible to distinguish genetic predisposition to react strongly to stress from environmentally determined variations in sensitivity. Thus, we cannot theorize about the relative contributions of each factor. We can, however, get a close-up view of how children react to a range of experimentally imposed environmental stressors; and further, see whether children who come from affective environments characterized diagnostically by high levels of conflict and distress, might show heightened sensitivity. Such appears to be the case. Childhood affective psychopathology should be a fruitful area for future research on environment-gene interaction. It is likely that both heredity and environment operate to a significant degree in producing the heightened reactivity to stress. Our focus has been on identifying some of the environmental factors because these utlimately might be amenable to intervention and prevention techniques. We may, for example, be able to teach parents to modify affective child-rearing techniques or teach the child requisite social skills at an early age, possibly through the use of peer tutors.

Study Two: Children of Unipolar Parents

Sample and Methods. In the next phase of research we asked whether children with a unipolar depressed parent would show patterns of socioemotional functioning similar to or different from those of children from bipolar families. Unipolar depression is not marked by the highs or manic behavior that characterizes bipolar depression. In this sample, mothers with unipolar depression were studied. As with the bipolar sample, none had been hospitalized for affective illness during the lifetime of the child. Diagnosis of the mothers again were based on SADS-L diagnostic interviews and DSM-III criteria. Twenty-three mothers were diagnosed as having unipolar depression (major or minor unipolar depression, past or current) and sixteen control mothers received diagnoses of normal. Mothers' reports were used to ascertain that fathers were free of serious affective psychopathology.

The group of children in this sample was exposed to a less extensive battery of procedures than the bipolar sample: They participated in the laboratory sessions at age two, and we report here on assessments of their peer relations and reactions to experimental simulations in the first two sessions. In other words, the procedures here were identical to those used in the laboratory portion of the first study.

Results and Discussion. Because these data have not yet been reported in the published literature, the descriptive data and inferential statistics associated with the significant findings are provided in this section. Sex differences did not appear at levels beyond that which would have been expected by chance. Therefore, findings reported are for the two sexes combined.

Aggression/Antisocial Behavior. Children with a unipolar depressed mother did not tend to show such overtly maladaptive patterns of aggression as did the children from bipolar families. Levels of aggressive behavior toward the adult experimenter following the frustration task did not differ for children from unipolar *(UD)* versus control *(C)* groups. However, different patterns of emotionality emerged. Children from the depressed (proband) group smiled more at the experimenter who imposed the frustration ($\bar{X}_{UD} = .52$, S.D. $= .51$, $\bar{X}_C = .12$, S.D. $= .34$, $F(1,37) = 7.34$, $p < .01$). Either they were less likely to take the event seriously, treating it as a game, or — more likely — they were trying to appease the unfamiliar adult. Children from the two groups differed significantly on some measures of aggression toward peers. Children with a unipolar depressed mother were less likely than controls to engage in acts of physical aggression, ($\bar{X}_{UD}$ = 1.35, S.D. = 1.82, $\bar{X}_C$ = 2.75, S.D. = 2.41, F (1,37) = 4.28, p < .05 for frequency of physical aggression and $\bar{X}_{UD}$ = 36.2 seconds, S.D. = 39.9, $\bar{X}_C$ = 8.8 seconds, S.D. = 18.8, F (1,37) = 8.37, p < .01 for time in physical aggression) or acts of intense aggression toward their playmates ($\bar{X}_{UD}$ = .74, S.D. = .96, $\bar{X}_C$ = 1.75, S.D. = 1.91, F (1,37) = 4.73, p < .05). When proband children were victims of aggression, they were somewhat more likely to show distress than control children ($\bar{X}_{UD}$ = 37.4, S.D. = 23.2, $\bar{X}_C$ = 24.2, S.D. = 25.0, F (1,37) = 2.85, p < .10). In contrast, children from control families tended to show more emotionality (particularly distress) when they, themselves were aggressing ($\bar{X}_{UD}$ = 30.2, S.D. = 27.8, $\bar{X}_C$ = 47.3, S.D. = 22.9, F (1,37) = 4.13, p < .05).

Altruism/Prosocial Behavior. In most respects, children of unipolar depressed parents and the control group showed very similar prosocial orientations. They showed similar levels of prosocial behavior toward playmates. In response to distress simulations, levels of total altruism toward mother, unfamiliar adult, and infant were comparable. Within subcategories of altruism, children with depressed mothers were somewhat more likely to use direct helping as a technique ($\bar{X}_{UD}$ = .30, S.D. = .47, $\bar{X}_C$ = .06, S.D. = .25, F (1,37) = 3.52, p < .075), while children of control mothers were more likely to try to distract or disengage the victim from the distress. For example, some controls tried to move the person into very unrelated activities; others tried to indicate that the problem would end soon ($\bar{X}_{UD}$ = .09, S.D. = .29, $\bar{X}_C$ = .38, S.D. = .50, F (1,37) = 5.19, p < .03). Children with a unipolar depressed mother also showed high levels of preoccupation during the simulations of distress ($\bar{X}_{UD}$ = .96, S.D. = .98, $\bar{X}_C$ = 1.81, S.D. = .98, F (1,37) = 7.23, p < .01); and they showed somewhat more positive affect to the unfamiliar adult ($\bar{X}_{UD}$ = .83, S.D. = .78, $\bar{X}_C$ = .37, S.D. = .72, F (1,37) = 3.37, p < .075) during the simulations of distress.

Social Interactions and Emotionality. There were differences in the patterns of social interactions of children from the proband and control groups, indicated in a statistical interaction of a diagnostic group with experimental situation (F (8,296) = 2.19, p < .05). When children first came into the play setting, the children with depressed mothers actually engaged in more sociable behavior toward their playmates than controls, but during exposure to the fight between the adults, there was a significant drop in their peer play: In the period preceding the adult fight, $\bar{X} = 4.30$, S.D. = 1.14, while in the period during the fight, $\bar{X} = 2.96$, S.D. = 1.02. The play of children from the control group was not similarly disrupted, $\bar{X} = 3.56$, S.D. = 1.03 preceding the fight and $\bar{X} = 3.31$, S.D. = 1.30 during the fight. During the remaining periods of peer play, levels of social interaction did not differ reliably for children with unipolar depressed mothers and children from control families. There is a suggestion here that disturbances in emotional tone may be responsible for the momentary inhibition of social interaction: During the fight between the adults, children from the proband group showed substantially higher levels of distress ($\bar{X}_{UD} = 5.70$, S.D. = 2.08, $\bar{X}_C = 4.25$, $F(1,37) = 5.45$, $p < .025$). Ratings of children's overall levels of distress across sessions, however, showed children of unipolar mothers as more contained in their expressions of distress ($\bar{X}_{UD} = 4.91$, S.D. = 1.00, $\bar{X}_C = 5.75$, S.D. = 1.61, $F(1,37) = 4.02$, $p < .05$).

To summarize, children with a unipolar depressed mother looked different, as a group, from children of control families. The former were especially sensitive to issues regarding physical and psychological harm that might befall another person. These proband children were less likely to engage in activities that might potentially bring physical injury to their playmates. They also became more preoccupied and upset when exposed to conflict and distress in others. This heightened emotionality sometimes momentarily disrupted their own social interactions. Children from control families on the other hand, were more inclined to turn away from others' problems. Their prosocial efforts in the same situations more often took the form of guiding the victim away from a problem rather than attempting to deal with it directly. Children with a unipolar depressed parent, at times, appeared already to be suppressing certain emotional tendencies. They were particularly polite in the face of frustration and seemed to make deliberate use of positive emotions to cope with some stressful situations.

Study Groups Compared. This composite portrait of a child of a unipolar depressed mother shows some commonalities with the predominant patterns shown by children from bipolar homes. Both groups of children showed signs of preoccupation or hypersensitivity toward the distress of others. Both showed signs of emotional disturbance following exposure to psychological stressors. But there were important differences as well, with the children of unipolar mothers appearing less profoundly upset and considerably more affectively controlled. Children of bipolar parents, in contrast, sometimes impressed researchers as less giving, more inappropriately aggressive, and more disregulated. It is important to bear in mind that not all children with an affectively ill parent showed problems and some children with normal parents showed problems. Also, there was a considerable range in the severity of apparent disturbance and levels of socioemotional competence in each of the groups of children studied. In particular, some children with depressed mothers looked very troubled, others appeared to be well socialized.

Future Research Directions

The discovery of atypical patterns of social and emotional functioning in offspring of depressed parents, already identifiable when children are just past infancy, are, to our knowledge, the first such reported data of this kind. Some of the early response dispositions of these children might represent manifestations or precursors of depression. This capacity of young children to be so influenced by their parent's affective state has implications that may alter theories and clinical practice. However, several questions remain unanswered by the research. These are questions that require a developmental psychopathological research perspective in order to be fully addressed. A major issue concerns which of the problem areas in socioemotional functioning identified in these children at risk will coalesce into diagnosable disturbances and which will disappear, which of the patterns are nonnormative but also nonpathological, and which predispositions might actually reflect superior functioning. Longitudinal research is currently being conducted to address some of these issues. The children described in this chapter will be seen again at ages five to six. They will be exposed to a series of challenging situations to assess their social competencies and vulnerabilities. Each child will also receive formal psychiatric assessments. We will then analyze the patterns of relations between early and later levels of socioemotional functioning to determine which early patterns may be precursors or prototypes of later depression.

More specifically, we will attempt to construct individual profiles of children that will reflect a continuum of emotional disturbance during the early years. For example, children who characteristically became enmeshed in other's problems, but who show few, if any, depressive symptoms, might constitute one level of disturbance. Children who were galvanized by the distress of others and who also showed other problems in modulation of emotion and impulse control might reflect a second level of difficulty. Still more problematical might be the children who showed the above disturbances and who were insecurely attached to the caregiver and unable to be comforted by her in times of stress. By following these different sets of children longitudinally we can then study how different constellations of symptoms or areas of concern do or do not culminate in later, diagnosable affective disturbance.

One reason for adopting the perspective of developmental psychopathology is to begin to provide more normative data on adaptive socioemotional functioning during the years of childhood. A useful research strategy that derives from this approach, and one that we have adopted here, is to compare children who are and who are not considered to be at risk for emotional disturbance. In other words, normal children from normal homes provide the baseline data on normal development, and deviations from this norm can be used to assess psychopathology. This approach can be helpful in identifying children at the extremes, as we have seen in the current research. For example, young children who virtually never show concern for another person, who rarely engage in social interaction, who become overly upset by and perseverate on other people's problems, who are unable to resolve conflicts directly, and so on, can be viewed both as displaying nonnormative responses and as exhibiting potential indicators of psychopathology. The point at which atypical behaviors and emotions qualify as deviant or symptomatic is less readily answerable.

Consider, for example, the meaning of the low levels of physical aggression found in children with a unipolar depressed parent. This could reflect relative inability to engage in normal rough-and-tumble play. In the animal literature, rough-and-tumble play is sometimes described as a mechanism for promoting assertiveness, competence, and social cohesion between animals. However, in humans the willingness to refrain from hurting others might reflect the early development of a higher level internalized norm or value regarding consideration for others. Obviously, a certain amount of aggression is adaptive, necessary, and hence normal in one sense, but ultimately, survival of our species and our civilizations will require lower levels of aggression. There appears to be a need in most societies to invest more in understanding the origins and control of aggression. In the meantime, there may be costs to the individual who does not fit the cultural norm of readiness to hurt others. Whether this should be labeled as psychopathological is another question.

Other aspects of the early sensitivities of children of unipolar depressed mothers also are open to alternative interpretations. Clinicians (for example, Miller, 1981) have commented on the frequency with which children of depressed parents assume a caregiver role; further, these children often become therapists as adults, presumably because of their highly developed, early sensitivity to others' needs. Such heightened sensitivity, however, could also reflect empathy gone awry which, in turn, might be a precursor of depression. Children from normal homes showed a greater tendency to deny distress. Again, while this may be seen as normative, it does not necessarily reflect ideal emotional functioning.

The caregivers in these particular unipolar and bipolar samples differed not only in type of depressive illness, but also in the severity of their problems. Many of the women who received diagnosis of unipolar depression were quite functional: They were sensitive, attuned to and able to express their feelings. Their children appeared similarly sensitive. Some of these unipolar mothers were more distressed and the bipolar sample of parents, in particular, showed notable difficulties. The problems in their children also appeared more serious and less ambiguous in their interpretation.

As a group, the bipolar parents expressed considerable concern that they would transmit illness to their offspring. These parents had been apprised of the literature on intergenerational patterns and had been told that the illness might be hereditary. If parents believe that the process of transmission is genetically determined, and thus view it as inevitable and uncontrollable, premature labeling of the child can help to ensure future difficulty (Lord, 1982). On the other hand, the belief that out-of-control, hostile, manic, or sad feelings are not one's fault may help the parent to relinquish strong guilt feelings that may be undermining their interactions with the child. Similarly, environmental explanations also may produce the belief that the problems are difficult to overcome or, conversely, that change is possible. In the bipolar sample we saw extremes of parenting that reflected these different beliefs. One mother had established a compensatory, cognitive enrichment program for her child. The mother approached the task with overwhelming intensity, providing chronic overstimulation to the child, causing the learning environment to become aversive. Another mother, when asked to play with her child as part of an experimental procedure, indicated that she did not know how. With a great deal of encouragement, she was able to help create a climate for play and to participate in it with her child.

Some Therapeutic Suggestions. In some families with serious disturbance, problems in social and emotional functioning were identified in both the parents and the children. Therapeutic regimens that would help to draw both parents and children into social interactions with other, more functional families, could prove useful. Seriously depressed parents could, thus, be encouraged and helped to spend time with parents who are not currently experiencing difficulties. This would follow the lines of programs in which "model" parents are trained to help adolescent parents, abusive parents, and so on.

In addition to constructing social relationships and environments for such families at risk, it is also possible to encourage them to extend their own social networks. Such a venture would not be without its own problems. Often the more affectively disturbed caregivers have difficulty in establishing and maintaining social relationships. When they do establish social ties, they may tend to gravitate toward other people with affective problems (similar to the process of assortative mating). We observed, for example, a tendency for depressed mothers to associate with other depressed mothers. If an affectively ill parent has chosen an affectively ill or otherwise disturbed spouse, and they in turn choose friends with similar problems an expanded depressogenic environment is fashioned. The children grow up playing with the children of the depressed friends and hence there are multiple opportunities for contagion or disregulation of emotion as well as for other kinds of problems. The negative implications of growing up in such an expanded (manic) depressive social network is vividly portrayed in autobiographic form (Hayward, 1977). Hayward describes both the specific disturbances in family processes and the special stimulation and opportunities that may sometimes derive from growing up with emotionally unusual, but also creative and talented, parents.

Research on offspring of depressed parents provides a unique opportunity for studying disregulation of affect as well as the onset—if it occurs—of depression in the children. Recent offspring studies have not been uniform in reporting deleterious effects of exposure to an affectively ill parent. For example, Sameroff and others (1982) have reported that children of neurotically depressed mothers have more problems than children with psychotic parents. Kauffman and others (1979) describe some children of psychotic parents as "super kids." Some studies, including ours, find many of the children to be well socialized, and not particularly aggressive; while other studies (Hops and others, 1983) find high rates of negative, oppositional behavior in children with depressed parents. Differences across studies may reflect, among other things, variations in (1) the severity of the diagnosed illness, (2) the instruments used to assess depression, (3) the particular type of depression and symptoms, (4) how the depression is manifested in parent-child interaction, and (5) the child behaviors measured. The inconsistencies do testify to the complexity of the phenomenon being studied. Depression in parenting may create problems for children or it may create special opportunities or it may do both. The challenge for future research is to begin to elucidate the etiology of these problems and the associated paradoxes.

Conclusion

At the beginning of this chapter we outlined several variables hypothesized to be responsible for depression. In addition to these factors, which will require continued investigation within developmental frameworks, we believe there are still other key concepts to be studied in the etiology of depression. We need to know more about the developmental processes by which feelings of responsibility for one's own distress, preoccupation with the distress of others, and inability to deal with personal despair begin to converge to create levels of sadness that become overwhelming and impervious to comfort and social support. The main feature that distinguishes depression from less enduring mood states is its pervasiveness. The depressed person is not well able to deny or turn away from distress. We have identified a parallel phenomenon in young children of depressed parents. Nor is the depressed person readily capable of self-comfort or receiving comfort from others. Disturbances in sleeping and eating patterns in depressed adults may, for example, represent primitive and ultimately ineffective attempts to self-comfort. Thus, it becomes important to begin to identify the mechanisms by which children learn (1) the ability to deny (at some adaptive level) or turn away from sadness and (2) the capacity to be comforted or consoled when distress cannot and should not be denied. The ability to adaptively let go of pain and suffering and to give and receive comfort appropriately should mitigate against depression. The etiology of these coping mechanisms merits investigation: The land of tears is, indeed, a mysterious place. Research, however, can help to clear away some of the secrecy surrounding depression in childhood.

References

Akiskal, H., and McKinney, W. "Overview of Recent Research in Depression: Integration of Ten Conceptual Models into a Comprehensive Clinical Frame." *Archives of General Psychiatry,* 1975, *32,* 285–305.

American Psychiatric Association. *Diagnostical and Statistical Manual of Mental Disorders.* (3rd ed.) Washington, D.C.: American Psychiatric Association, 1980.

Anthony, E. J. "The Influence of a Manic-Depressive Environment on the Developing Child." In E. J. Anthony and T. Benedek (Eds.), *Depression and Human Existence.* Boston: Little, Brown, 1975.

Beardslee, W., Bemporad, J., Keller, M., and Klerman, G. "Children of Parents with Major Affective Disorder: A Review." *American Journal of Psychiatry,* 1983, *140* (7), 825–832.

Beck, A. *Cognitive Therapy and the Emotional Disorders.* New York and Scarborough, Ontario: Times Mirror, 1979.

Bibring, E. "The Mechanism of Depression." In P. Greenacre (Ed.), *Affective Disorders.* New York: International Universities Press, 1953.

Block, J. H. *The Child Rearing Practices Report.* Berkeley: Institute of Human Development, University of California, 1965.
Bowlby, J. *Attachment and Loss.* Vol. III: *Loss, Sadness, and Depression.* New York: Basic Books, 1980.
Cicchetti, D. "The Emergence of Developmental Psychopathology." *Child Development,* 1984, *55,* 1-7.
Crook, T., Raskin, A., and Eliot, J. "Parent-Child Relationships and Adult Depression." *Child Development,* 1981, *52,* 950-957.
Cytryn, L., McKnew, D. H., Bartko, J. J., Lamour, M., and Hamovit, J. "Offspring of Patients with Affective Disorders, II." *Journal of the American Academy of Child Psychiatry,* 1982, *21,* 389-391.
Davenport, Y. B., Adland, M. L., Gold, P. W., and Goodwin, F. K. "Manic-Depressive Illness: Psychodynamic Features of Multigenerational Families." *American Journal of Orthopsychiatry,* 1979, *49,* 24-35.
Davenport, Y. B., Zahn-Waxler, C., Adland, M. L., and Mayfield, A. "Early Childrearing Practices in Bipolar Families." *American Journal of Psychiatry,* 1984, *141,* 230-235.
de Saint Exupéry, A. *The Little Prince.* New York: Harcourt Brace Jovanovich, 1943.
Emde, R. N. "Toward a Psychoanalytic Theory of Affect." In S. I. Greenspan and G. H. Pollock (Eds.), *The Course of Life: Psychoanalytic Contributions Toward Understanding Personality Development.* Vol. I: *Infancy and Early Childhood.* Washington, D.C.: National Institute of Mental Health, 1980, 63-83.
Fieve, R. R., Mendlewicz, J., and Fleiss, J. L. "Manic-Depressive Illness: Linkage with the Hg Blood Group." *American Journal of Psychiatry,* 1973, *130,* 1355-1359.
Gaensbauer, T. J., and Hiatt, S. "Facial Communication of Emotion in Early Infancy." In N. Fox and R. J. Davidson (Eds.), *Affective Development: A Psychobiological Perspective.* Hillsdale, N.J.: Erlbaum, 1984.
Goodman, S. H. "Young Children of Severely Emotionally Disturbed Mothers." Presentation at the conference of The Society for Research in Child Development, Detroit, Mich., April 1983.
Gross, W. B., and Siegel, P. B. "Socialization by Humans Reduces Health Risks Among Chickens." *American Journal of Veterinary Research,* 1982, *43,* 2010-2012.
Grunebaum, H., Cohler, B. J., Kauffman, C., Gallant, D. "Children of Depressed and Schizophrenic Mothers." *Child Psychiatry and Human Development,* 1978, *8,* 219-228.
Hammon, C., and Hiroto, D. "Psychosocial Study of Children of Depressed Parents." Paper presented to the Yale Vulnerability Consortium, New Haven, Conn., March 1983.
Hayward, B. *Haywire.* New York: Knopf, 1977.
Hops, H., Biglan, A., Sherman, L., Arther, J., and Friedman, L. S. "Direct Observation Study of Family Processes in Maternal Depression." Poster session: Studies of Depression in Child and Adult Populations, American Psychological Association, Anaheim, Calif., September 1983.
Kandell, E. "Changes in the Brain Produced by Learning." Presentation at a symposium on the Science of the Brain, American Psychiatric Association, Toronto, Alberta, Canada, May 1982.
Kashani, J., Husain, A., Shekim, W., Hodges, K., Cytryn, L., and McKnew, D. H. "Current Perspectives on Childhood Depression: An Overview." *American Journal of Psychiatry,* 1981, *38* (2), 143-153.
Kauffman, C., Grunebaum, H., Cohler, B., and Gamer, E. "Superkids: Competent Children of Psychotic Mothers." *American Journal of Psychiatry,* 1979, *11,* 1398-1402.
Lord, C. "Psychopathology in Early Development in the Young Child." *Reviews of Research.* Vol. 3. National Association for the Education of Young Children, Washington, D.C., 1982.

Mayo, J. A., O'Connell, R. A., and O'Brien, J. D. "Families of Manic-Depressive Patients: Effects of Treatment." *American Journal of Psychiatry,* 1979, *136* (12), 1535-1539.

Meyersberg, H. A., and Post, R. M. "A Holistic Developmental View of Neural and Psychological Processes." *British Journal of Psychiatry,* 1979, *135,* 139-155.

Miller, A. *Prisoners of Childhood. The Drama of the Gifted Child and the Search for the True Self.* New York: Basic Books, 1981.

Musick, J., Klehr, K., Cohler, B., and Clark, R. "Results of a Five-Year Intervention Program for Young Children at Risk for Psychopathology." Presentation at a conference of The Society for Research in Child Development, Detroit, Mich., April 1983.

Orvaschel, H., Weissman, M. M., and Kidd, K. K. "Children and Depression: The Children of Depressed Parents; The Childhood of Depressed Patients; Depression in Children." *Journal of Affective Disorders,* 1980, *2,* 1-16.

Pansepp, J. "The Psychobiology of Prosocial Behaviors: Separation Distress, Play, and Altruism." In C. Zahn-Waxler, E. M. Cummings, and R. Iannotti (Eds.), *The Social and Biological Origins of Altruism and Aggression.* Cambridge, England: Cambridge University Press, in press.

Poznanski, E. O., Carroll, B. J., Bemejas, M. C., Cook, S. C., and Grossman, J. A. "The Dexamethasone Suppression Test in Prepubertal Depressed Children." *American Journal of Psychiatry,* 1982, *139,* 321-324.

Provence, S. "Depression in Infancy?" *Zero to Three* (Bulletin of the National Center for Clinical Infant Programs), 1983, *3* (4), 1-4.

Puig-Antich, J. "Major Depression and Conduct Disorder in Pre-Puberty." *Journal of the American Academy of Child Psychiatry,* 1982, *21* (2), 118-128.

Radke-Yarrow, M., Kuczynski, L., Zahn-Waxler, C., Cytryn, C., McKnew, D. H., Cummings, E. M., and Iannotti, R. "Affective Disorders and Affective Development in Normal Families and Families with Affective Disorders." National Institute of Mental Health Research Protocol, Clinical Project Number 79-M-123, 1982.

Rolf, J. E. "Peer Status and the Directionality of Symptomatic Behavior: Social Competence Predictors of Outcome for Vulnerable Children." *American Journal of Orthopsychiatry,* 1976, *46,* 74-88.

Rutter, M., and Garmezy, N. "Developmental Psychopathology." In P. Mussen (Ed.), *Handbook of Child Psychology.* Vol. IV: *Socialization, Personality and Social Development.* (4th ed.) New York: Wiley, 1984.

Sameroff, A. J., Seifer, R., and Zax, M. "Early Development of Children at Risk for Emotional Disorder." *Monographs of the Society for Reserach in Child Development,* 1982, *47,* 1-71.

Seligman, M. E. P., and Maier, S. F. "Failure to Escape Traumatic Shock." *Journal of Experimental Psychology,* 1967, *74,* 1-9.

Spitz, R. A. "Anaclitic Depression: An Inquiry into the Genesis of Psychiatric Conditions in Early Childhood, II." *Psychoanalytic Study of the Child,* 1946, *2,* 313-324.

Spitzer, R. L., and Endicott, J. *Schedule for Affective Disorders and Schizophrenia-Lifetime Version (SADS-L).* New York: Biometrics Research Division, New York State Psychiatric Institute, 1978.

Spivack, G., and Shure, M. *Social Adjustment of Young Children: A Cognitive Approach to Solving Real-Life Problems.* San Francisco: Jossey-Bass, 1974.

Sroufe, L. A., and Rutter, M. "The Domain of Developmental Psychopathology." *Child Development,* 1984, *55,* 17-29.

Stern, D. "Ongoing Research on Developmental Psychopathology of Depressive Phenomena." *Zero to Three* (Bulletin of the National Center for Clinical Infant Programs), 1983, *3* (4), 1-4.

Watson, M. W., and Fischer, K. W. "A Developmental Sequence of Agent Use Late in Infancy." *Child Development,* 1977, *48,* 828-836.

Weintraub, S., Prinz, R. J., and Neale, G. M. "Peer Evaluations of the Competence of Children Vulnerable to Psychopathology." *Journal of Abnormal Child Psychology,* 1978, *6,* 461-473.

Zahn-Waxler, C., Chapman, M., Cummings, E. M., and Cytryn, L. "Cognitive and Social Development in Infants and Toddlers with a Bipolar Parent." Paper presented at the annual meeting of the American Academy of Child Psychiatry, Washington, D.C., 1982.

Zahn-Waxler, C., Cummings, E. M., McKnew, D. H., and Radke-Yarrow, M. "Altruism, Aggression, and Social Interactions in Young Children with a Manic-Depressive Parent." *Child Development,* 1984a, *55,* 112-122.

Zahn-Waxler, C., McKnew, D. H., Cummings, E. M., Davenport, Y., and Radke-Yarrow, M. "Problem Behaviors and Peer Interactions of Young Children with a Manic-Depressive Parent." *American Journal of Psychiatry,* 1984b, *141,* 236-240.

Carolyn Zahn-Waxler conducts research at the Laboratory of Developmental Psychology at the National Institute of Mental Health.

E. Mark Cummings conducts research at the Laboratory of Developmental Psychology at the National Institute of Mental Health.

Ronald J. Iannotti conducts research at the Laboratory of Developmental Psychology at the National Institute of Mental Health.

Marian Radke-Yarrow heads the Laboratory of Developmental Psychology at the National Institute of Mental Health.

Index

A

Aboud, F. E., 61, 78
Abramson, L. Y., 51, 55
Achenbach, T. M., 43, 45, 55
Adland, M. L., 103
Aggression, by offspring, 91–92, 95–96, 99
Ainsworth, M. D. S., 14, 25, 35, 55
Akiskal, H. S., 7, 25, 82, 102
Altruism, by offspring, 92, 96
Ambrosini, P. J., 26
American Psychiatric Association, 6, 25, 55, 59, 62, 63, 77, 88, 102
Anderson, J. C., 78
Anhedonia, developmental view of, 36
Anthony, E. J., 29, 55, 82, 87, 102
Antisocial behavior, by offspring, 91–92, 95–96
Arend, R. A., 57
Arther, J., 103

B

Bartko, J. J., 103
Beardslee, W., 84, 102
Beck, A. T., 30, 39, 55, 56, 60, 62, 77, 79, 83, 102
Behavioral systems, and psychopathology, 14–15
Bemejas, M. C., 104
Bemporad, J. R., 37, 38, 39, 40, 51, 55, 60, 78, 102
Bibring, E., 60, 78, 82, 102
Biglan, A., 103
Bischof, N., 14, 25
Blau, S., 57
Blehar, M., 55
Block, J. H., 93, 103
Boag, L. C., 56, 79
Bowlby, J., 14, 15, 25, 82, 103
Braunwald, K., 27
Bressler, E., 5n
Bromley, D. B., 51, 56
Brown, F., 56
Brown, M. B., 78

Brumback, R. A., 30, 38, 55
Bruss-Saunders, E., 80
Buckler, J. M. H., 66, 78
Bunney, W. E., 56
Burke, P. M., 27
Burton, N., 52, 56, 60, 79

C

Campbell, S. B., 75, 78
Cantwell, D. P., 59, 61, 76, 78
Carlson, G. A., 41, 55, 59, 61, 76, 78
Carlson, V., 27
Carnap, R., 18, 25
Carroll, B. J., 57, 104
Chadwick, D., 57
Chambers, W. J., 26, 45, 57, 79
Chandler, M., 13, 19, 22, 26
Chapman, M., 105
Child Behavior Checklist, 45
Children: in adolescence, 41–42; of depressed parents, 81–105; in infancy, 37–38; preschool, 38–39, 88–98; school-aged, 39–41, 43–54, 63–77
Children's Depression Inventory (CDI), 44, 46–47, 54
Children's Depression Rating Scale (CDRS): advantages of, 53–54; in assessment battery, 44–45, 46–47, 52, 53; and symptoms, 48, 49
Cicchetti, D., 1–27, 31, 32–33, 35, 50, 51, 55–56, 82, 103
Clark, C. J., 27
Clark, R., 104
Clarkson, S. E., 78
Cognitive development, depression related to, 62, 64–66, 67, 68, 72, 76–77
Cohler, B. J., 103, 104
Combinations Task (CT), 64, 65, 67
Commins, S., 38, 56
Competence, role of, in depression, 8
Conners, C. K., 60, 78
Conservation-withdrawal, by infants, 38
Cook, S. C., 57, 104
Costello, C. G., 53, 56
Crook, T., 83, 103

107

Crouse-Novak, M. A., 79
Cummings, E. M., 2-3, 27, 87-105
Cytryn, C., 104
Cytryn, L., 26, 29, 31, 50, 56, 61, 78, 86, 103, 104, 105

D

Damon, W., 40, 51, 56, 61, 70, 78
Davenport Y. B., 27, 82, 83, 86, 87, 93, 103, 105
Davies, M., 26, 79
Depression, childhood: acuteness and chronicity of, 68; in adolescence, 41-42; and age, 45-48, 73-74; anaclitic, 37; assessment of, 44-45; background on, 5-6; biological correlates of, 7; and chi-squares tests, 73; children at risk for, 81-105; classification of, 37-43; clinical evaluation and diagnosis of, 64; and demographic data, 45; developmental perspective on, 35-37; developmental progression of, 29-58; and developmental stage, 67-73; diagnostic criteria for, 6-7, 30-31, 35-36; diathesis for, 9; discussion of findings on, 49-54, 73-77; empirical study of, 43-54; etiology of, 7, 19-23, 82-83, 102; expression of, and developmental stage, 59-80; findings on, 45-49, 66-73; and guilt, 51; and hopelessness, 51; in infants, 37-38; literature review on, 37-43; log-linear model analysis of, 69-70; masked, 30, 39, 50, 70, 74; method of studying, 43-45, 62-66; organizational approach to, 10-15; in preschool children, 38-39, 88-98; prevalence of, 73; research on, 59-60, 82-86; research strategies for, 83-86; risk factors for, 19-23; in school-aged children, 39-41, 43-54, 63-77; and self-esteem, 50-51; sequelae of, 7-8; stepwise discriminant analyses of, 70-73; subjects with, 43-44, 63-64; and suicidal ideation, 51-52; symptoms of, 47-48, 86-87; transactional model of, 5-27; verbalized feelings of, 50; views of, 29-30. See also Psychopathology
de Saint Exupéry, A., 81, 103
Dettmers, R., 81n
Development: concept of, 10-11, 32; explanatory power of, 75-77; issues in assessment of, 74-75; normal, concept of, 11; normal, knowledge of, 8-9, 34-35; stage of, and expression of depressive disorders, 59-80
Developmental perspective: axioms of, 32-33; on childhood depression, 35-37; and children at risk, 81-105; on classification of depression, 37-43; defining, 32-37; empirical study of, 43-54; goals of, 82; history of, 60-61; implications of, 1, 34-35; and nosology, 33-34; and progression of depression in girls, 29-58; and transactional model, 5-27; usefulness of, 6-10
Diagnostic and Statistical Manual-III (DSM-III), 6-7, 31, 45, 59, 63, 64, 88, 95
Diagnostic Interview for Children and Adolescents (DICA), 45
Dietz-Schmidt, G., 55
Dixon, W. J., 69, 78
Doob, L. W., 51, 56

E

Edelbrock, C. S., 45, 55
Eliot, J., 103
Elkind, D., 73, 78
Emde, R. N., 83, 103
Emotionality, by offspring, 92, 96-97
Endicott, J., 27, 80, 104
Engel, G., 18, 25, 37, 38, 56
Engelman, L., 78

F

Feinberg, T. L., 79
Fieve, R. R., 86, 103
Finkelstein, R., 79
Fischer, K. W., 89, 104
Fisher, P., 52, 57
Flavell, J. H., 39, 56
Fleiss, J. J., 103
Frane, J. W., 78
Friedman, L. S. 103
Friedman, R. J., 80

G

Gaensbauer, T. J., 8, 25-26, 83, 103
Gallant, D., 103
Garner, E., 103

Garber, J., 2, 29–58
Garmezy, N., 29n, 81, 82, 104
Gaylin, W., 60, 78
Gelman, R., 62, 78
George, C. E., 12, 26
Girich, Y. P., 38–39, 40, 41, 42, 51, 52, 53, 58
Girls, developmental perspective on depression among, 43–54
Gittelman, R., 7, 26
Gittelman-Klein, R., 30, 56
Glasberg, R., 61, 78
Glaser, K., 30, 37, 50, 56, 61, 70, 78
Gold, P. W., 103
Goodman, S. H., 84, 103
Goodnow, J., 65, 78
Goodwin, F., K, 103
Gorman, B. S., 61, 80
Gottesman, I., 16, 26
Graham, P., 57
Graham, S., 51, 58
Greenhill, L. L., 57
Greenspan, S. I., 33, 34, 35, 56
Gross, W. B., 94, 103
Grossman, J. A., 104
Grunebaum, H., 85, 103
Guilt, and depression, 51
Guze, S. B., 45, 57

H

Halpern, F., 26, 79
Hamilton, M., 44, 56
Hamilton Depression Rating Scale, 44
Hammon, C., 84, 103
Hamovit, J., 103
Hanlon, C., 26, 79
Harmon, R., 26
Hart, D., 40, 51, 56, 61, 70, 78
Harter, S., 22, 26
Hayward, B., 101, 103
Heisler, A. B., 38, 56
Herjanic, B., 45, 56
Herjanic, M., 56
Herzog, D. B., 60, 61, 78
Hiatt, S., 83, 103
Hierarchical motility, and psychopathology, 13
Hill, M. A., 78
Hiroto, D., 84, 103
Hodges, K. K., 26, 103
Hoetz, R., 79
Holism, and psychopathology, 11–12

Hollingshead, A. B., 63, 78
Holzman, P., 5n
Hopelessness, and depression, 51
Hops, H., 84, 101, 103
Husain, A., 26, 103

I

Iannotti, R. J., 2–3, 87–105
Inamdar, S. C., 61, 80
Inhelder, B., 65, 79
Interpersonal Reasoning Tasks (IRT), 64–65, 66, 67
Interview Schedule for Children (ISC), 64, 69

J

Jacobson, E., 60, 78
Jaquette, D., 57, 80
Jenrich, R. I., 78
Joffe, W. G., 14, 26, 38, 57
Jones, M., 29n

K

Kandell, E., 94, 103
Kanner, L., 29, 56
Kaplan, B., 10, 12, 13, 26, 27
Kashani, J. H., 5, 26, 73, 78, 82, 103
Katz, M. M., 80
Kauffman, C., 85, 101, 103
Keller, M., 102
Kidd, K. K., 104
Klehr, K., 104
Klerman, G., 102
Kovacs, M., 2, 30, 35, 44, 51, 56, 59–80, 84
Krawiec, V., 26
Kuczynski, L., 104

L

Laird, J. D., 51, 57
Lamour, M., 103
Lefkowitz, M. M., 52, 56, 60, 79
Lipinski, J., 5n
Livesly, W. J., 51, 56
Lord, C., 100, 103
Lourie, R. S., 56
Lupartkin, W., 26

M

McCauley, E. A., 27
McConville, B. J., 40-41, 42, 51, 53, 56, 61, 79
McGee, R. O., 78
McKinney, W. T., Jr., 7, 25, 82, 102
McKnew, D. H., 26, 27, 50, 56, 61, 78, 103, 104, 105
Mahler, M. S., 29, 30, 57
Maier, S. F., 83, 104
Main, M., 12, 26
Makita, K., 60, 61, 73, 79
Malmquist, C. P., 29n, 37, 50, 57, 60, 61, 79
Marx, N., 57
Matas, L., 32, 57
Mayfield, A., 103
Mayo, J. A., 86, 104
Meehl, P. E., 5n, 9, 106, 26, 29n
Mendlewicz, J., 103
Mental pain, defined, 14
Meyersberg, H. A., 83, 94, 104
Microgenesis, and psychopathology, 12-13
Miller, J., 10, 26
Minneapolis Public School System, 29n, 43
Minnesota, University of, 29n
Mohr, D. M., 65, 67, 79
Mullener, N., 51, 57
Musick, J., 84, 104
Myers, J. K., 43, 58

N

National Institute of Mental Health, 5n, 29n, 59n, 88
Neale, G. M., 105
Novacenko, H., 26
Nover, R. A., 56

O

O'Brien, J. D., 104
O'Connell, R. A., 104
Offspring of depressed parents: affective problems among, 81-105; of bipolar parents, 86-95; comparison of, 97-98; conclusion on, 102; findings on, 91-97; home assessments of, 88-89; laboratory assessments of, 89-91; longitudinal research on, 98; research needed on, 98-101; research strategy for, 84-85; samples of, 88, 95; therapeutic suggestions for, 100-101; of unipolar parents, 95-98
Organizational approach, to psychopathology, 10-15
Orthogenetic principle, concepts in, 12-13; and developmental perspective, 32; polarities of, 13-14; and psychopathology, 11-14
Orvaschel, H., 58, 84, 104
Outcome, process distinct from, 12

P

Padian, N., 58
Pakaluk, M., 5n
Panksepp, J., 94, 104
Pap, A., 18, 26
Parent Form of the Children's Depression Inventory (P-CDI), 44, 46-47, 54
Parents. See Offspring of depressed parents
Paulauskas, S. L., 2, 59-80
Pearce, J. B., 49, 57
Penick, E. C., 58
Perel, J. M., 26
Personal Identity Interview (PII), 64, 65, 67
Piaget, J., 13, 26, 37, 57, 61, 65, 75, 76, 79
Pittsburgh, University of, 63
Pogge-Hesse, P., 8, 24, 25, 33
Pollock, M., 79
Post, R. M., 83, 94, 104
Poznanski, E. O., 38, 44, 52, 57, 73, 79, 84, 104
Precursor studies, 85-86
Preskorn, S. H., 60, 79
Prinz, R. J., 105
Process, outcome distinct from, 12
Prosocial behavior, by offspring, 92, 96, 99
Provence, S., 83, 104
Psychopathology: and behavioral systems, 14-15; concept of, 11; continuity in, 34; developmental view of, 33; diathesis-stress model of, 16-17; early experience model of, 15-16; main-effects model of, 15-16; organizational approach to, 10-15; and orthogenetic

principle, 11-14; prediction, origin, and manifestations of, 33; vulnerability model of, 17-18
Pubertal stage, depression related to, 61, 64, 67, 68, 69, 71-72
Puig-Antich, J., 6, 7, 26, 31, 45, 57, 60, 75, 79, 84, 104
Purohit, A. P., 56, 79

R

Radke-Yarrow, M., 2-3, 27, 87-105
Raskin, A., 103
Rathbun, J. M., 60, 61, 78
Redman, L. D., 57
Reichsman, F., 37, 38, 56
Renshaw, D. C., 52, 57
Research Diagnostic Criteria (RDC), 6-7, 59
Rie, H. E., 5, 26, 29, 30, 51, 57, 60, 61, 79
Risk factors: mechanism-specific and general, 22-23; in transactional model, 19-23
Robins, A. J., 78
Robins, E., 27, 45, 57, 80
Rochlin, G., 29, 30, 57, 60, 79
Rolf, J. E., 85, 104
Rubin, K. H., 62, 79
Rutman, J., 58
Rutter, M., 8, 26, 27, 31, 32, 33, 42, 43, 50, 57, 58, 73, 79, 81, 82, 104

S

Sachar, E. J., 26, 79
Sameroff, A., 13, 19, 22, 26, 101, 104
Sandler, J., 14, 26, 38, 57
Santostefano, S., 33, 57
Saussure, R. de, 29, 57
Schedule for Affective Disorders and Schizophrenia for children (Kiddie-SADS), 45
Schedule of Affective Disorders and Schizophrenia-Lifetime Version (SADS-L), 88, 95
Schneider-Rosen, K., 1-27, 31, 32, 33, 35, 50, 51, 56
Schuyler, D., 80
Schwartz, R. M., 61, 80
Secunda, S. K., 73, 80
Seifer, R., 104
Self-esteem, and depression, 50-51
Seligman, M. E. P., 55, 83, 104
Sellars, W. S., 18, 27
Selman, R. L., 51, 57, 65, 66, 75, 80
Shaffer, D., 51-52, 57
Shantz, C. U., 61, 80
Shea, C., 26
Sherman, L., 103
Shields, J., 16, 26
Shure, M., 88, 104
Siegel, P. B., 94, 103
Silva, P. A., 78
Simonds, J. F., 73, 78
Siomopoulos, G., 61, 80
Shekim, W. O., 26, 103
Social interactions, by offspring, 92, 96-97
Somatosexual maturity, depression related to, 61, 64, 67, 68, 69, 71-72
Sommer, B. B., 50, 58
Spitz, R. A., 37, 38, 58, 83, 104
Spitzer, R. L., 6, 27, 59, 80, 104
Spivack, G., 88, 104
Spring, B., 17, 27
Sroufe, L. A., 8, 19, 27, 29n, 31, 32, 33, 57, 58, 81, 104
Stern, D., 83, 104
Stiller, R. L., 26
Strober, M., 41, 55
Suicidal ideation, and depression, 51-52
Sullivan, L., 58
Sylvester, C. E., 8, 27

T

Tabrizi, M. A., 26, 79
Tanner, J. M., 64, 66, 67, 80
Teasdale, J. D., 55
Tellegen, A., 29n
Thompson, J., 79
Tizard, J., 57
Toolan, J. M., 30, 58, 70, 80
Toporek, J. D., 78
Trabasso, T., 61, 80
Transactional model: analysis of, 5-27; conclusion on, 23-25; described, 18-23; factors in, 20-22; proposals relevant to, 15-18; risk factors in, 19-23

U

Ushakov, G. K., 38-39, 40, 51, 52, 53, 58

V

Verducci, J., 59n
Von Bertalanffy, L., 9, 10, 18, 25
Vulnerability model of psychopathology, 17–18

W

Waddington, C. H., 13, 19, 22, 27
Wall, S., 55
Walton, L. A., 78
Washburn Child Guidance Clinic, 29n
Waters, E., 8, 27, 55
Watson, M. W., 89, 104
Wechsler Intelligence Scale for Children-Revised (WISC-R), 43, 63
Weinberg, W. A., 30, 38, 55, 58
Weiner, B., 51, 58
Weintraub, S., 85, 88, 105
Weissman, M. M., 43, 54, 58, 104
Weitzman, E. D., 79
Weller, E. B., 79
Weller, R. A., 79
Welner, Z., 74, 80
Werner, H., 10, 11, 12, 27, 32, 58
Wessman, A. E., 61, 80
Weston, B., 60, 75, 79
Wheatt, T., 56
Whitmore, K., 57
Williams, S., 78
Wilson, A., 37, 38, 39, 40, 51, 55
Wylie, R. C., 51, 58

Y

Yale, W., 57

Z

Zahn-Waxler, C., 2–3, 8, 27, 87–105
Zax, M., 104
Zrull, J. P., 38, 57, 73, 79
Zubin, J., 17, 27

U.S. POSTAL SERVICE
STATEMENT OF OWNERSHIP, MANAGEMENT AND CIRCULATION
(Required by 39 U.S.C. 3685)

1. TITLE OF PUBLICATION: New Directions for Child Development	A. PUBLICATION NO. 4 9 4 0 9 0	2. DATE OF FILING: 9/30/84
3. FREQUENCY OF ISSUE: quarterly	A. NO. OF ISSUES PUBLISHED ANNUALLY: 4	B. ANNUAL SUBSCRIPTION PRICE: $35 inst/$25 indv

4. COMPLETE MAILING ADDRESS OF KNOWN OFFICE OF PUBLICATION *(Street, City, County, State and ZIP Code) (Not printers)*
433 California St., San Francisco (SF County), CA 94104

5. COMPLETE MAILING ADDRESS OF THE HEADQUARTERS OR GENERAL BUSINESS OFFICES OF THE PUBLISHERS *(Not printers)*
433 California St., San Francisco (SF County), CA 94104

6. FULL NAMES AND COMPLETE MAILING ADDRESS OF PUBLISHER, EDITOR, AND MANAGING EDITOR *(This item MUST NOT be blank)*

PUBLISHER *(Name and Complete Mailing Address)*
Jossey-Bass Inc., Publishers, 433 California St., San Francisco, CA 94104

EDITOR *(Name and Complete Mailing Address)*
William Damon, Dept. of Psychology, Clark Univ. Worcester, MA 01610

MANAGING EDITOR *(Name and Complete Mailing Address)*
William Henry, Jossey-Bass Publishers, 433 California St., S.C. CA 94104

7. OWNER *(If owned by a corporation, its name and address must be stated and also immediately thereunder the names and addresses of stockholders owning or holding 1 percent or more of total amount of stock. If not owned by a corporation, the names and addresses of the individual owners must be given. If owned by a partnership or other unincorporated firm, its name and address, as well as that of each individual must be given. If the publication is published by a nonprofit organization, its name and address must be stated.) (Item must be completed.)*

FULL NAME	COMPLETE MAILING ADDRESS
Jossey-Bass Inc., Publishers	433 California St., S.F., CA 94104
For names and addresses of stockholders, see attached list.	

8. KNOWN BONDHOLDERS, MORTGAGEES, AND OTHER SECURITY HOLDERS OWNING OR HOLDING 1 PERCENT OR MORE OF TOTAL AMOUNT OF BONDS, MORTGAGES OR OTHER SECURITIES *(If there are none, so state)*

FULL NAME	COMPLETE MAILING ADDRESS
Same as #7	

9. FOR COMPLETION BY NONPROFIT ORGANIZATIONS AUTHORIZED TO MAIL AT SPECIAL RATES *(Section 411.3, DMM only)*
The purpose, function, and nonprofit status of this organization and the exempt status for Federal income tax purposes *(Check one)*

☐ (1) HAS NOT CHANGED DURING PRECEDING 12 MONTHS
☐ (2) HAS CHANGED DURING PRECEDING 12 MONTHS

10. EXTENT AND NATURE OF CIRCULATION

	AVERAGE NO. COPIES EACH ISSUE DURING PRECEDING 12 MONTHS	ACTUAL NO. COPIES OF SINGLE ISSUE PUBLISHED NEAREST TO FILING DATE
A. TOTAL NO. COPIES *(Net Press Run)*	1595	1593
B. PAID CIRCULATION 1. SALES THROUGH DEALERS AND CARRIERS, STREET VENDORS AND COUNTER SALES	165	103
2. MAIL SUBSCRIPTION	506	506
C. TOTAL PAID CIRCULATION *(Sum of 10B1 and 10B2)*	671	609
D. FREE DISTRIBUTION BY MAIL, CARRIER OR OTHER MEANS SAMPLES, COMPLIMENTARY, AND OTHER FREE COPIES	133	120
E. TOTAL DISTRIBUTION *(Sum of C and D)*	804	729
F. COPIES NOT DISTRIBUTED 1. OFFICE USE, LEFT OVER, UNACCOUNTED, SPOILED AFTER PRINTING	791	864
2. RETURN FROM NEWS AGENTS	0	0
G. TOTAL *(Sum of E, F1 and 2—should equal net press run shown in A)*	1595	1593

11. I certify that the statements made by me above are correct and complete

[Signed] John R. Ward, Vice-President

Ministry of Education, Ontario
Information Centre, 13th Floor,
Mowat Block, Queen's Park,
Toronto, Ont. M7A 1L2